THE ALKAINE DIET FOR DADDY AND SON

2 Books in 1: For Beginners: The Ultimate Guide of Alkaline Herbal Medicine for permanent weight loss, Understand pH with 200+ Anti Inflammatory Recipes Book! Plant-Based Meals Are Included!

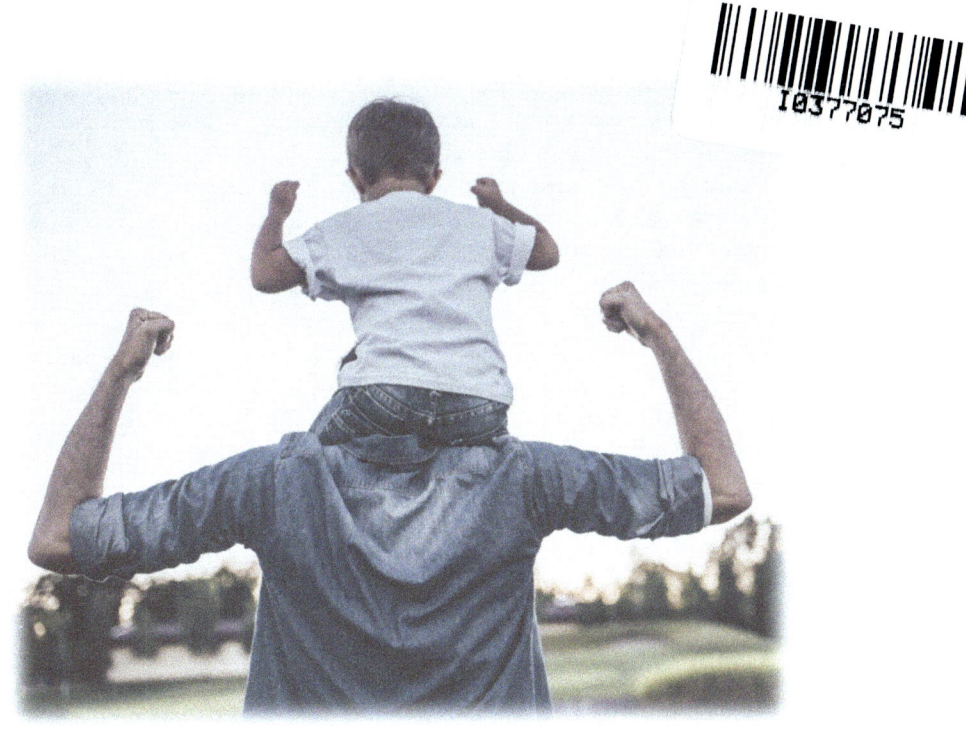

By

Laura Green

TABLE OF CONTENT

PART 1- INTRODUCTION 8
BREAKFAST & SMOOTHIES 13
1) Baked walnut oatmeal 14
2) Banana waffles 14
3) Savoury sweet potato waffles 15
4) Oatmeal and fruit pancakes 15
5) Frozen banana breakfast bowl 15
6) Chia seed and blueberry cobbler 15
7) Quick and easy granola bars 16
8) Alkaline Blueberry Spelt Pancakes 16
9) Alkaline blueberry muffins 16
10) Meal of crispy quinoa 17
11) Coconut pancakes 17
12) Quinoa Porridge 17
13) Amaranth porridge 17
LUNCH 18
14) Wakame and pepper salad 19
15) Green salad of orange and avocado 19
16) Green salad with cucumbers and mushrooms 19
17) Chickpea, vegetable and fonio salad 19
18) Avocado and chickpea salad 20
19) Amaranth, cucumber and chickpea salad 20
20) Avocado and rocket salad with citrus fruits 21
21) Avocado salad and spelt noodles 21
22) Lettuce salad with basil 21
23) Cabbage and sprout salad 21
24) Watercress and cucumber salad 22
25) Watercress and orange salad 22
26) Mushroom and olive salad 22
27) Asparagus salad with cashew sauce 23
28) Sweet potato salad with jalapeno sauce 23
29) Green pineapple salad 24
30) Sweet Peach Tahini Salad 24
31) Pasta salad with red lentils and vegetables 24
32) Fennel and carrot salad 25
33) Tofu and watermelon salad 25
34) Spinach and strawberry salad with lemon vinaigrette 25
35) Rainbow salad with citrus mango dressing 26
36) Roasted cabbage and beetroot salad 26
37) Spelt pasta with avocado 26
38) Lettuce and mushroom burger with basil 27
39) Zoodles with tomato sauce and avocado 27
40) Mushroom and pepper fajitas 27
41) Chickpea and mushroom sausages 28
42) Mushroom and kale ravioli 28
43) Lettuce wrap and courgette hummus 29

44)	Apple and pumpkin burger by Butternut	29
45)	Cabbage and avocado	29
46)	Courgette bacon	30
47)	Mushroom and pepper fritters	30
48)	Chickpea, pepper and mushroom curry	30
49)	Spelt noodles with peppers and mushrooms	31
50)	Okra and tomato curry	31
51)	Sage mushrooms in the oven	31
52)	Spelt pasta with Swiss chard	32
53)	Baked pumpkin and apples	32

DINNER..33

54)	Vegetarian stew	34
55)	Quinoa and lentil stew	34
56)	Black bean chili	34
57)	Kidney bean curry	35
58)	Green beans in a casserole	35
59)	Vegetarian cake	36
60)	Rice and lentil meatloaf	36
61)	Asparagus risotto	37
62)	Quinoa and chickpea salad	37
63)	Mixed vegetable soup	37
64)	Bean and barley soup	37
65)	Tofu and pepper stew	38
66)	Chickpea stew	38
67)	Lentils with cabbage	39
68)	Vegetarian Ratatouille	39
69)	Baked beans	39
70)	Barley Pilaf	40
71)	Vegetable and salmon kebabs	40
72)	Coconut curry with vegetables	40
73)	Spaghetti squash loaded	41
74)	Spicy pasta	41
75)	Stuffed peppers	41
76)	Baba Ganoush Pasta	42
77)	Broccoli bowl with cheese	42
78)	Green bean and lentil salad	42
79)	Vegetable soup	43
80)	South West Hamburger	43
81)	Courgette rolls with red sauce	44
82)	Meatless Taco Wraps	44
83)	Sesame and quinoa pilaf	45

SNACKs..46

84)	Aloo Gobi	47
85)	Chocolate Crunch Bars	47
86)	Walnut butter Bars	47
87)	Homemade Protein Bar	47
88)	Shortbread Coookies	48
89)	Coconut biscuits Chip	48
90)	Coconut Cookies	48

91)	Berry Mousse	48
92)	Coconut pulp Coookies	49
93)	Avocado Pudding	49
94)	Coconut Raisins cooookies	49
95)	Cracker Pumpkin Spice	49
96)	Spicy Toasted nuts	50

DESSERTS 51

97)	Cabbage and pineapple smoothie	52
98)	Green vegetable smoothie	52
99)	Avocado and spinach smoothie	53
100)	Cucumber smoothie	53
101)	Apple and ginger smoothie	53
102)	Blueberry smoothie with green tea	53
103)	Apple and almond smoothie	54
104)	Cranberry smoothie	54
105)	Berry and cinnamon smoothie	54
106)	Detoxifying berry smoothie	54
107)	Pink smoothie	55
108)	Green apple smoothie	55

PART 2- INTRODUCTION TO THE ALKALINE DIET 56

BREAKFAST & SMOOTHIES 62

109)	Chocolate quinoa porridge	63
110)	Buckwheat porridge with walnuts	63
111)	Fruity oatmeal	64
112)	Baked walnut oatmeal	64
113)	Almond fritters	64
114)	Amaranth porridge	65
115)	Banana porridge	65
116)	Courgette muffins	65
117)	Tofu stew with vegetables	65
118)	Courgette fritters	66
119)	Quinoa with pumpkin	66
120)	Avocado toast	66
121)	Frozen banana breakfast bowl	66

LUNCH 67

122)	Vegetarian lettuce rolls	68
123)	Oatmeal, tofu and spinach burger	68
124)	Hamburger with beans, nuts and vegetables	69
125)	Avocado stuffed with tofu and broccoli	69
126)	Brussels sprouts with walnuts	70
127)	Broccoli with cabbage	70
128)	Mushrooms with parsley	70
129)	Garlic broccoli	71
130)	Broccoli with peppers	71
131)	Spicy okra	71
132)	Spicy cauliflower	72
133)	Aubergine curry	72
134)	Lemon cabbage with shallots	72
135)	Vegetables with apple	73

136)	Cabbage with apple	73
137)	Asparagus with herbs	73
138)	Vegetarian Kabobs	74
139)	Tofu with Brussels sprouts	74
140)	Tofu with broccoli	74
141)	Tempeh in tomato sauce	75
142)	South West Stuffed Sweet Potatoes	75
143)	Coconut cauliflower with herbs and spices	75
144)	Quinoa and Brussels sprouts salad	76
145)	Mango and jicama salad	76
146)	Asparagus and roasted mushroom salad	76
147)	Thai green salad	76
148)	Avocado and quinoa salad	77
149)	Caprese salad	77
150)	Tagliatelle with pumpkin and broccoli salad	77
151)	Broccoli and mandarin salad	77
152)	Spinach and mushroom salad	78
153)	Broccoli, asparagus and quinoa salad	78
154)	Root salad	78
155)	Lush summer salad	78
156)	Salad of sea vegetables and algae	78
157)	Rainbow salad	79
158)	Rocket salad with basil	79
159)	Green cucumber and rocket salad	79
160)	Strawberry and dandelion salad	80
161)	Wakame and pepper salad	80
DINNER		81
162)	Carrot and potato stew with herbs	82
163)	Berry and mint soup	82
164)	Potato and broccoli soup	83
165)	Lush pepper soup	83
166)	Cabbage and yellow onion soup	83
167)	Wild rice, mushroom and leek soup	84
168)	Pear and ginger soup	84
169)	Asparagus and artichoke soup	84
170)	Carrot and celery soup	85
171)	Creamy clam chowder with mushrooms	85
172)	Bok choy soup, broccolini and brown rice	85
173)	Apple and sweet pumpkin soup	86
174)	Tomato and carrot soup with lemon	86
175)	Courgette and avocado soup with basil	86
176)	Courgette, spinach and quinoa soup	87
177)	Easy Cilantro Lime Quinoa	87
178)	Spinach Quinoa	87
179)	Healthy broccoli Asparagus Soup	88
180)	Creamy Asparagus Soup	88
181)	Spicy Eggplant	88
182)	Brussels Sprouts and carrots	89
183)	Matured Cajun Zucchini	89

184)	Fried cabage	89
185)	Tofu Curry	89
186)	Cauliflower with sauce	90
187)	Zucchini Noodles	90
188)	Buckwheat Porridge	90
189)	Vegetable soup	91
190)	Lentil and spinach soup	91
191)	Vegetarian stew	91

SNACKs 92

192)	Alka-Goulash fast	93
193)	Pea risotto	93
194)	Satisfying lunch smoothie Alka	93
195)	Alkaline pizza bread	94
196)	Alkaline-filled avocado	94
197)	Alkaline potato salad	94
198)	Almonds with sautéed vegetables	95
199)	Alkaline sweet potato mash	95
200)	Mediterranean peppers	95
201)	Tomato and avocado sauce with potatoes	95
202)	Alkaline beans and coconut	96
203)	Alkaline vegetable lasagne	96
204)	Aloo Gobi	97

DESSERTS 98

205)	Pumpkin smoothie	99
206)	Red fruit and vegetable smoothie	100
207)	Kale smoothie	100
208)	Green tofu smoothie	100
209)	Grape and chard smoothie	100
210)	Matcha Smoothie	101
211)	Banana smoothie	101
212)	Strawberry smoothie	101
213)	Raspberry and tofu smoothie	101
214)	Mango smoothie	102
215)	Pineapple smoothie	102
216)	Cabbage and pineapple smoothie	102

AUTHOR BIBLIOGRAPHY 104
CONCLUSIONS 106

© Copyright 2021 - All rights reserved.

The content contained within this book may not be reproduced, duplicated or transmitted without direct written permission from the author or the publisher.

Under no circumstances will any blame or legal responsibility be held against the publisher, or author, for any damages, reparation, or monetary loss due to the information contained within this book. Either directly or indirectly.

Legal Notice:

This book is copyright protected. This book is only for personal use. You cannot amend, distribute, sell, use, quote or paraphrase any part, or the content within this book, without the consent of the author or publisher.

Disclaimer Notice:

Please note the information contained within this document is for educational and entertainment purposes only. All effort has been executed to present accurate, up to date, and reliable, complete information. No warranties of any kind are declared or implied. Readers acknowledge that the author is not engaging in the rendering of legal, financial, medical or professional advice. The content within this book has been derived from various sources. Please consult a licensed professional before attempting any techniques outlined in this book.

By reading this document, the reader agrees that under no circumstances is the author responsible for any losses, direct or indirect, which are incurred as a result of the use of information contained within this document, including, but not limited to, — errors, omissions, or inaccuracies.

PART 1- INTRODUCTION

Let's start with a bit of review of our chemistry lessons and remember what pH is. A simple definition is how much concentration of hydrogen ions there is in our body. The acronym pH is an abbreviation for "hydrogen potency." The "p" stands for "potent" or the German word for power, and "H" stands for the symbol for the element hydrogen. The pH scale ranges from 1 to 14. Seven is neutral. A pH below seven is acidic. Solutions that have a pH above seven are alkaline.

To have good health, our bodies must be somewhat alkaline. The pH of our blood and other cellular fluids should be around a pH between 7.365 and 7.45. It is essential to understand that pH levels vary significantly throughout the body. Some parts will be acidic, while others will be alkaline. There is no set level. For example, our stomach is loaded with hydrochloric acid, which gives it a pH of between 2 and 3.5. This makes it very acidic. It needs to be this acidic to break down the foods we consume and kill harmful bacteria. Our saliva has a pH between 6.8 and 7.3. Our skin has a pH between 4 and 6.5. This acts as a protective barrier from the environment. Our urine has a pH that ranges from alkaline to acidic. It all depends on what you eat.

The most critical measure is the pH of your blood. It needs to stay in a very narrow range between 7.365 and 7.45. This may sound simple, but instead of operating on a mathematical scale, our pH operates on a logarithmic scale in multiples of ten. This means that it will take ten times the amount of alkalinity to neutralize an acid. A pH of five will be 100 times more acidic than a pH of seven. A pH of four will be 1,000 times more acidic. Does this help you understand?

Don't start stressing about being in or out of this range. Remember that our bodies are pretty good at regulating the pH of our blood. However, our bodies do not "find" the balance. It has many parts that do, and it keeps the blood pH between 7.365 and 7.45 at all times. If you make poor lifestyle and food choices, your body works harder to maintain balance. If you want to address inflammation and acidity in your body by changing your food choices to more alkaline foods, this will help balance your system and bring your body back to its best vitality.

BLOOD pH

You know that the body is constantly working to maintain healthy pH levels in your body. The tricky thing is that three fluids in the body are typically at slightly different pH levels. But overall, they're primarily controlled by the same things. So the first thing we're going to look at is blood pH.

The normal pH range for blood is 7.35 to 7.45. This means that blood is usually alkaline or basic by nature. However, compared to stomach acid, which is between 3 and 5.5, a significant difference can be seen. The stomach is supposed to be at this acid level to break down the food you eat. Ironically, if your stomach acid becomes more acidic or more essential, it can create the same symptoms of acid reflux, but that's another matter. This low pH helps you digest your food and destroys germs that may enter your stomach.

What can cause your blood pH to change or reach abnormal levels?

Health problems are usually the most common cause of your blood becoming too alkaline or acidic. In addition, a change in normal blood pH levels can signal a medical emergency or health condition. This may include:

- Poisoning
- Drug overdose
- Bleeding
- Shock
- Infection
- Gout
- Lung disease

- Kidney disease
- Heart disease
- Diabetes
- Asthma

Acidosis refers to when the blood pH level drops below 7.35 and begins to become too acidic. Alkalosis refers to when the blood pH level rises to more than 7.45 and becomes too alkaline. Two main organs work hard to help maintain normal pH levels in the blood:

- Kidneys - These organs work by removing acid through urine to excrete it.
- Lungs - These organs work by getting rid of carbon dioxide through breathing.

The different forms of blood alkalosis and acidosis depend significantly on the cause. However, the two leading causes are:

- Metabolic - These types of problems occur most often when the pH of the blood changes due to a problem with a condition in the kidneys.
- Respiratory - These types of problems occur most often when the blood pH changes due to a respiratory or pulmonary condition.

It is common for blood pH levels to be tested as part of a blood gas test. This type of test is also called an ABG test or arterial blood gas test. It works by measuring how much carbon dioxide and oxygen are in your blood. Your primary care doctor may choose to test your blood pH as a regular part of your annual health screenings or if you already have certain health conditions. Blood pH testing requires drawing blood with a needle. The lab will receive the blood sample and perform the test.

There are blood pH tests you can do at home by pricking your finger. These tests will not give you an accurate reading like a test in your doctor's office. Using a urine pH test will not show you the pH level of your blood, but it can let you know if something is wrong.

Let's take a moment to take a closer look at some reasons why your blood pH levels are moving outside of the normal range.

High blood pH, also known as alkalosis, occurs if your blood pH rises above the normal range. There are many reasons for high blood pH levels. For example, you may have a temporary increase in blood pH with simple illnesses. Certain foods can also cause your blood to become more alkaline. However, there are also more serious causes for this alkalosis that can create additional problems.

The first is fluid loss. Losing too much water can cause the pH levels in your blood to rise. This is because you also lose certain electrolytes in your blood, minerals, and salts when you lose water. These include potassium and sodium. In addition, diarrhea, vomiting, and sweating can cause you to lose excess fluids.

Medications and diuretics can also cause a person to urinate more often, leading to increased pH levels in the blood. Treatment for fluid loss requires making sure to take plenty of fluids and replacing electrolytes. Some sports drinks can be used for this purpose. Your doctor can also review your medications and stop those that may be causing fluid loss.

Next, kidney problems can cause high pH levels in the blood. The kidneys play an essential role in maintaining normal blood pH. Therefore, a kidney problem can cause a buildup of alkalinity in the blood. This is because the kidneys do not remove excess alkaline substances through the urine. For example, the kidneys may improperly filter bicarbonate in the blood. Medications can regulate this.

When there is acidosis in the blood, it can affect the functioning of every organ in the body. Low blood pH is a more common problem than high blood pH. Therefore, acidosis is often a warning sign of some health problem that is not being controlled.

Some health conditions can cause natural acids to build up in the blood. Some forms of acids that can end up lowering the pH of the blood include:

- Carbonic acid
- Hydrochloric acid
- Phosphoric acid
- Sulfuric acid
- Ketogenic acids
- Lactic acid

An improper diet can cause problems. Eating an unbalanced diet can create a temporary low pH level in the blood. Not eating enough or going for long periods without eating can produce more acid in the blood. Try to avoid eating too many acid-forming foods, which include:

- Grains - rice, pasta, bread, and flour
- fish
- Meat
- Eggs
- Poultry - turkey and chicken
- Dairy products - yogurt, cheese, and cow's milk

Balance your blood pH by eating more alkaline foods. These include dried, frozen, and fresh fruits and fresh, cooked vegetables more often. Stay away from fad or starvation diets. Instead, when you're trying to lose weight, do so healthily and safely by following a balanced diet.

Another cause of low blood pH levels is due to diabetic ketoacidosis. If you have diabetes, your blood can end up turning acidic if you don't properly regulate your blood sugar levels. Diabetic ketoacidosis occurs when your body can't make enough insulin or use it properly.

Insulin helps move sugar from the foods we eat to the cells in the body. This is where the body burns it as fuel. If insulin cannot be used, the body begins to break down the fat stored in the body for energy. This releases a wasted acid known as ketones. If the body cannot regulate this process, the acid will build up and trigger a low pH in the blood.

You must seek emergency care if your blood sugar level exceeds 300 milligrams per deciliter. If you suffer from any of the following symptoms, talk to your doctor:

- Confusion
- Stomach pain
- Shortness of breath
- Shortness of breath
- Vomiting or nausea
- Weakness or fatigue
- Frequent urination
- Excessive thirst

Diabetic ketoacidosis is most often a sign that diabetes is not being treated properly and is out of control. This can sometimes be the first sign of diabetes for some people. Making sure your diabetes is well treated will help keep your blood pH in balance. It may require a strict diet and exercise plan, insulin injections, and medications to stay healthy.

The third cause of low blood pH is metabolic acidosis. This is when low blood pH is caused by kidney disease or failure. This occurs when there is a kidneys failure to remove acids from the body through urination. This will increase the acids in the body and lower the pH of the blood.

The most common symptoms of metabolic acidosis include
- Heavy breathing
- Fast heartbeat
- Headaches
- Vomiting and nausea
- Loss of appetite
- Weakness and fatigue

Treatment for this problem often includes medications to help the kidneys work better, but a kidney transplant or dialysis is the only solution for severe cases. Dialysis works by cleansing the blood.

The final cause of low pH in the blood is respiratory acidosis. When the lungs are probably not working to remove carbon dioxide from the body quickly, blood pH levels drop. This will happen more often if a person has a chronic or severe lung condition, such as:
- Diaphragm disorders
- Chronic obstructive pulmonary disease
- Pneumonia
- Bronchitis
- Sleep apnea
- Asthma

People who are obese, have had surgery, or abuse opioid painkillers or sedatives are at increased risk of developing respiratory acidosis. In some cases, the kidneys can take over and remove excess blood acids through excretion. As a result, a person may need to receive extra oxygen and medications such as steroids and bronchodilators to help the lungs function correctly. In very severe cases, mechanical ventilation and intubation may be necessary for individuals with respiratory acidosis to bring the blood pH back to normal.

- Urine pH

The next type of pH we will examine is that of urine. Urine is composed of waste products, salts, and water that are excreted through the kidneys. The balance of these different compounds can affect the acidity level of the urine. According to the American Association for Clinical Chemistry, the average urine pH is 6.0, but it can range from 4.5 to 8.0. Any level below 5.0 is considered acidic urine, and any level above 8.0 is considered primary urine.

Sometimes different labs have different ranges on what they consider normal pH levels for urine. One of the main things that affect the pH of your urine is the things you eat. If you go to your doctor, he or she will often ask you what foods you ate before evaluating the results of a urine pH test.

If, before a test, you ate more acidic foods, your urine will be more acidic. The same is true if you have eaten more alkaline foods. If a person has extremely high pH levels in their urine, meaning it is more alkaline, it could be the result of problems such as
- Urinary tract infections
- Kidney stones
- Other kidney-related disorders

A person may also have high pH levels in their urine if they have had prolonged vomiting. This is because vomiting causes the body to get rid of stomach acid, which causes the body's fluids to become more essential.

When urine is acidic, it creates an environment conducive to kidney stones. When urine is acidic, it can also be a sign of several severe medical conditions, such as:
- Hunger
- Diarrhea
- Diabetic ketoacidosis

As you'll notice, much of this is the same as blood pH levels. Some medications can affect the pH of the urine. Sometimes doctors will ask the patient to discontinue certain medications the day or night before doing a urinalysis.
- Saliva pH

The final pH we will look at is the pH of saliva. The usual range of saliva pH is 6.2 to 7.6. The things you drink and eat can change the pH of your saliva.

Just like any other area of your body, your mouth needs to maintain a balanced pH. Saliva pH levels can drop below 5.5 when you've had a lot of acidic drinks. In this case, the acids in your mouth begin to break down the enamel on your teeth.

If the enamel on your teeth becomes too thin, the dentin will be exposed. This can end up causing discomfort when you consume sugary, cold, or hot drinks. Just to give you an example of foods and drinks that can do this, here are some numbers:
- Cherries have a pH of 4
- American cheese has a pH of 5
- White wine has a pH of 4
- Soft drinks have a pH of 3

It's easy to spot unbalanced pH levels in your saliva. Some of the most common indicators are:
- Tooth decay
- Sensitivity to cold or hot drinks or foods
- Persistent bad breath

If you want, you can also test the pH of your saliva. The pH of your saliva can be tested: you'll need to find pH strips. Once you have the strips, here's what you need to do:
- Make sure you don't eat or drink anything for at least two hours before the test.
- Let your mouth fill with saliva and then swallow or spit it out.
- Let your mouth fill with saliva again, and then put a small amount on one of your pH strips.
- The strip will then react to your saliva. It will change color based on how alkaline or acidic your saliva is. The container the pH strips came with should show a color chart. Place your strip next to the chart to match the colors and determine the pH level of your saliva.

To make sure the pH of your saliva stays balanced, you need to eat foods that are in a healthy pH range. It is also to continue absorb essential vitamins and minerals. There are some more effective ways to make sure the pH of your saliva stays balanced.
- Stay away from sugary drinks. If you must drink them, try to swig them and chase them with water. Sipping sugary beverages for an extended period does more damage.
- Limit black coffee. Adding a little cream, unsweetened, can help reduce the acidity of coffee.
- Avoid brushing your teeth immediately after consuming high-acid beverages such as beer, wine, cider, juice, or soda. These types of beverages soften tooth enamel.
- Chew sugar-free gum after consuming any beverage or food. Chewing gum causes your mouth to produce more saliva and helps bring your pH level back to normal. It is also believed that xylitol can prevent bacteria from sticking to your tooth enamel. Always remember to keep yourself hydrated, so be sure to drink plenty of water.

BREAKFAST & SMOOTHIES

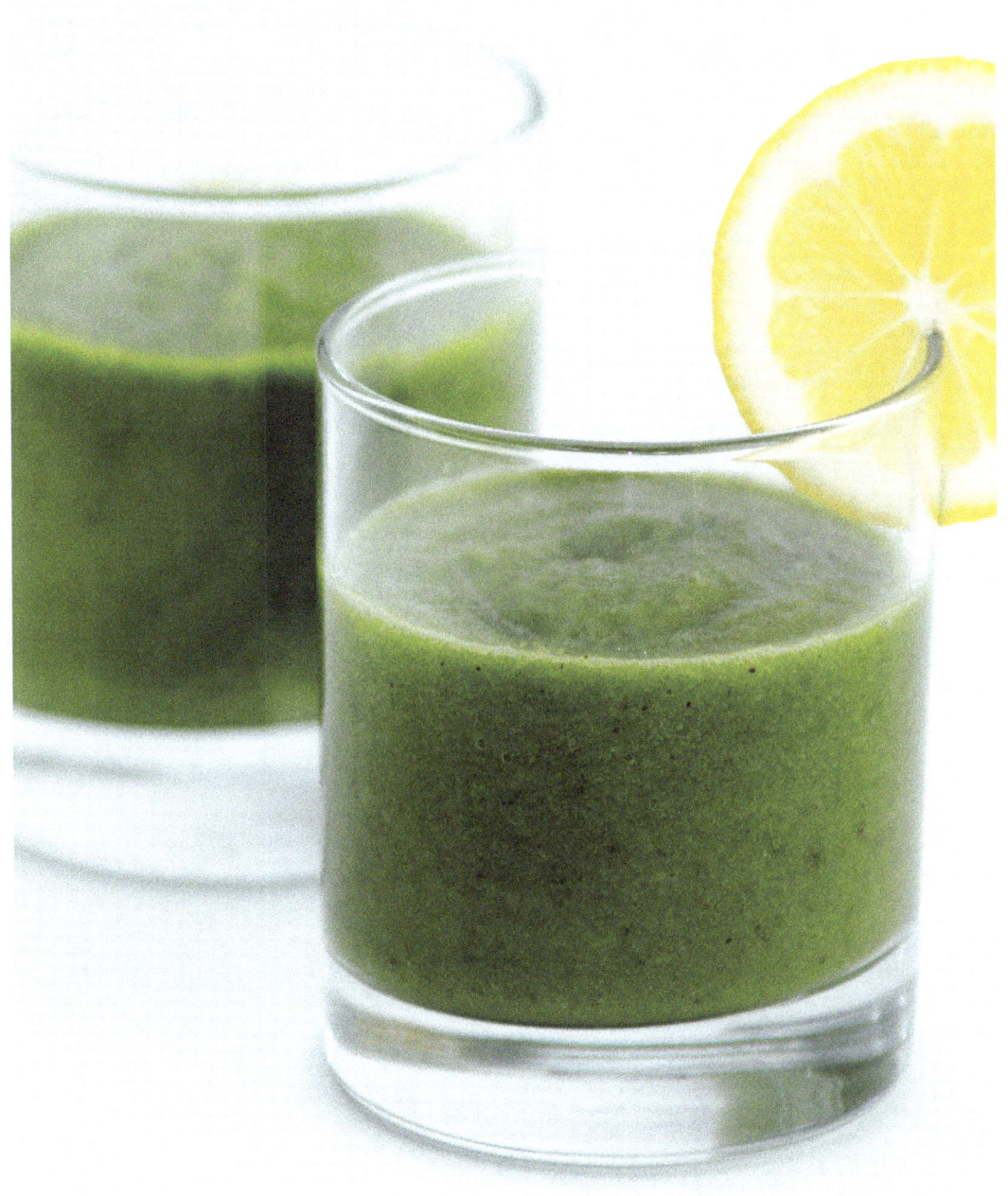

1) Baked walnut oatmeal

Preparation time: 15 minutes **Cooking time:** 45 minutes **Portions: 5**

Ingredients:
- ✓ 1 tablespoon linseed meal
- ✓ 3 tablespoons of alkaline water
- ✓ 3 cups unsweetened almond milk
- ✓ ¼ cup maple syrup
- ✓ 2 tablespoons coconut oil, melted and cooled
- ✓ 2 teaspoons of organic vanilla extract

Ingredients:
- ✓ 1 teaspoon cinnamon powder
- ✓ 1 teaspoon organic baking powder
- ✓ ¼ teaspoon of sea salt
- ✓ 2 cups old rolled oats
- ✓ ½ cup almonds, chopped
- ✓ ½ cup walnuts, chopped

Directions:
- ❖ Lightly grease an 8x8-inch baking dish. Set aside.
- ❖ In a large bowl, add the flaxseed meal and water and beat until well combined. Set aside for about 5 minutes.
- ❖ In the bowl of the flax mixture, add the remaining ingredients except the oats and nuts and mix until well combined.
- ❖ Add the oats and nuts and stir gently to combine.
- ❖ Place the mixture in the prepared baking tin and spread it out in an even layer.
- ❖ Cover the baking tray with plastic wrap and refrigerate for about 8 hours.
- ❖ Preheat the oven to 350 degrees F. Place a wire rack in the centre of the oven.
- ❖ Remove the tray from the refrigerator and let it rest at room temperature for 15-20 minutes.
- ❖ Remove the plastic film and mix the oatmeal mixture well.
- ❖ Bake for about 45 minutes.
- ❖ Remove from the oven and set aside to cool slightly.
- ❖ Serve hot.

2) Banana waffles

Preparation time: 15 minutes **Cooking time:** 20 minutes **Portions: 5**

Ingredients:
- ✓ 2 tablespoons of linseed flour
- ✓ 6 tablespoons of warm alkaline water
- ✓ 2 bananas, peeled and mashed

Ingredients:
- ✓ 1 cup creamy almond butter
- ✓ ¼ cup whole coconut milk

Directions:
- ❖ In a small bowl, add the linseed flour and warm water and whisk until well combined.
- ❖ Set aside for about 10 minutes or until the mixture becomes thick.
- ❖ In a medium bowl, add the bananas, almond butter and coconut milk, mix well.
- ❖ Add the flax meal mixture and stir until well combined.
- ❖ Preheat the waffle iron and grease it lightly.
- ❖ Place the desired amount of batter in the preheated waffle iron.
- ❖ Cook for about 3-4 minutes or until the wafers turn golden brown.
- ❖ Repeat with the remaining mixture.
- ❖ Serve hot.

3) Savoury sweet potato waffles

Preparation time: 10 minutes   **Cooking time:** 20 minutes   **Portions: 2**

Ingredients:
- 1 medium sweet potato, peeled, grated and squeezed
- 1 teaspoon fresh thyme, chopped
- 1 teaspoon fresh rosemary, chopped

Ingredients:
- 1/8 teaspoon red pepper flakes, crushed
- Sea salt and freshly ground black pepper, to taste

Directions:
- Preheat the waffle iron and then grease it.
- In a large bowl, add all the ingredients and mix until well combined.
- Put ½ of the sweet potato mixture into the preheated waffle iron and bake for about 8-10 minutes or until golden brown.
- Repeat with the remaining mixture.
- Serve hot.

4) Oatmeal and fruit pancakes

Preparation time: 10 minutes   **Cooking time:** 15 minutes   **Portions: 3**

Ingredients:
- 1 cup rolled oats
- 1 medium banana, peeled and mashed
- ¼-½ cup unsweetened almond milk
- 1 tablespoon organic baking powder

Ingredients:
- 1 tablespoon organic apple cider vinegar
- 1 tablespoon agave nectar
- ½ teaspoon organic vanilla extract
- ½ cup of fresh blackberries

Directions:
- Place all the ingredients except the blackberries in a large bowl and mix until well combined.
- Gently add the blackberries.
- Set the mixture aside for about 5-10 minutes.
- Preheat a large non-stick frying pan over medium-low heat.
- Add about ¼ cup of the mixture and with a spatula, spread into an even layer.
- Immediately, cover the pan and cook for about 2-3 minutes or until golden brown.
- Flip the pancake over and bake for a further 1-2 minutes or until golden brown.
- Repeat with the remaining mixture.
- Serve hot.

5) Frozen banana breakfast bowl

Preparation time: **Cooking time:**   **Portions: 1**

Ingredients:
- Chia seeds, hemp seeds, unsweetened coconut flakes, for garnish - optional
- Pumpkin seed protein powder, 4 tablespoons

Ingredients:
- Bananas, 2

Directions:
- Peel and then slice the bananas. Place them thinly in a freezer-safe container and freeze overnight.
- The next morning, add the bananas to a food processor and blend until a smooth, creamy consistency is achieved, much like that of soft-serve ice cream.
- Process the pumpkin protein powder through the bananas until it is just combined.
- Pour into a serving dish and add the desired toppings, if desired, and enjoy.

6) Chia seed and blueberry cobbler

Preparation time: **Cooking time:**   **Portions: 4**

Ingredients:
- Blueberry mixture -
- Chia seeds, 1 tablespoon
- Unrefined whole cane sugar, 2 tablespoons
- Blueberries, 2 c.
- Topping -
- Almond flour, .5 c.
- Sea salt, .25 teaspoon
- Vanilla pod powder, 1 teaspoon

Ingredients:
- A mixture of bicarbonate of soda and cream of tartar, 1.5 teaspoons
- Unrefined whole cane sugar, 2 tablespoons
- Melted coconut oil, 2 tablespoons
- Coconut milk, 4 tablespoons
- Oatmeal, .5 c.

Directions:
- Start by setting your oven to 350.
- To make the blueberries, mix the chia seeds, sugar and blueberries. Place the blueberry mixture in the bottom of four 4-ounce baking cups.
- To make the topping, mix together the salt, vanilla powder, baking powder, sugar, coconut oil, coconut milk, oatmeal and almond flour.
- Divide the blueberry topping between the four ramekins. You can leave the topping by spoonfuls, or you can spread it evenly over the blueberry mixture to create a complete crust.
- Bake the cobblers for 45 minutes, or until the topping has turned golden brown and everything is heated through. Enjoy.

7) Quick and easy granola bars

Preparation time: **Cooking time:** **Portions: 6**

Ingredients:
- Vanilla pod powder, .25 teaspoon
- Cinnamon spice, .25 teaspoon
- Sea salt, .25 teaspoon
- Coconut oil, 1 tablespoon

Directions:
- Place some parchment in the bottom of a 9x5 inch baking tin.
- Add the vanilla pod powder, cinnamon, salt, coconut oil, brown rice syrup, almond butter and oats to a food processor and blend until well combined.

Ingredients:
- Brown rice syrup, 2 tablespoons
- Almond butter, .5 c.
- Rolled quick oats, 1 c.

- Slide the dough into the baking tray and press it down into an even dough, making sure it is well compressed. Refrigerate the bars for 15-20 minutes, or until they are completely firm.
- Cut the granola into six bars and enjoy. Store the leftovers in the fridge. At room temperature, they will become soft.

8) Alkaline Blueberry Spelt Pancakes

Preparation time: 6 mnutes.   **Cooking time:** 20 minutes.   **Portions: 3**

Ingredients:
- 2 cups of spelt flour
- 1 cup coconut Milk
- 1/2 cup Alkaline Water
- 2 tbsps. Grape sed Oil

Directions:
- Mix together in a whisk the spellated flower, agave, wheat sed oil, hemp seeds and moss5s together.
- To the menstruum, add 1 cup of sheep's milk and cologne until you get the consistency menstruum you like.

Ingredients:
- 1/2 cup Agave
- 1/2 cup Blueberries
- 1/4 teaspoon musk Sea

- Mash the blue into the batter.
- Heat over medium heat and then lightly coat with the cereal oil.
- Put the butter in the oven and let it cook for about 5 minutes on all sides.
- Serve and have fun.

9) Alkaline blueberry muffins

Preparation time: 5 Minutes.   **Cooking time:** 20 minutes.   **Portions: 3**

Ingredients:
- 1 cup of coconut milk
- 3/4 cup of Spelt Flour
- 3/4 Teff flour
- 1/2 cup Blueberries

Directions:
- Adjust the oven temperature to 365 degrees.
- Grate 6 regular-size muffin cups with muffin liners.
- In a bowl, mix the sea salt, moss, agave, nut milk and flour until liquid.

Ingredients:
- 1/3 cup of Agave
- 1/4 cup Sea Moss Gel
- 1/2 teaspoon coarse salt, ground salt, olive oil

- Then crimp in blueberries.
- Cover the muffins lightly with the wheat seeds.
- Pour in the batter of muffin.
- Bake for at least 30 minutes until golden brown.
- Serve.

10) Meal of crispy quinoa

Preparation time: 5 minutes **Cooking time:** 25 minutes. **Portions: 2**

Ingredients:
- 3 cups of nut milk coco
- 1 cup rinsed quinoa.
- 1/8 tsp. cinnamon powder

Directions:
- In a saucepan, your milk and bring to a boil over moderate heat.
- Add the milk and then soak it once more.
- Then leave to stand for at least 15 minutes over a medium heat until the milk has reduced.

Ingredients:
- 1 cup raspberry
- 1/2 coconut

- Being higher in the corner than in the middle of the world.
- Cook for 8 minutes until the milk is ready to use.
- Add the raspberry and coook the meal for 30 seconds.
- Serve enjoy.

11) Coconut pancakes

Preparation time: 5 minutes. **Cooking time:** 15 minutes. **Portions: 4**

Ingredients:
- 1 cup coconut flour
- 2 tbsps. Arrow root powder
- 1 tsp. baking powder

Directions:
- In a medium container, mix all the ingredients.
- Add the coconut milk and 2 tbsps. Del coconut oil and mix properly.
- In a frying pan, melt 1 tsp. of coco walnut oil.
- Pour a ladleful of batter into the container and then spread the batter evenly on a smooth surface.

Ingredients:
- 1 cup coco walnut milk
- 3 tbsps. Coconut oil

- Coook il form for a least 3 minutes on average heat until you becomes firm.
- Flip the pancake onto the other side and cook for a further 2 minutes until golden brown.
- Cook the pancakes in a microwave oven.
- Serve.

12) Quinoa Porridge

Preparation time: 5 minutes. **Cooking time:** 25 minutes. **Portions: 2**

Ingredients:
- 2 cups coco nut milk
- 1 cup rinsed quinoa.

Directions:
- In a saucepan, boil the nut milk at a high temperature.
- Add the quinoa to the milk and then bring the mixture to a boil.
- Then you let it sit for 15 mnutes on medium heat until the milk has reduced.

Ingredients:
- 1/8 tsp. ground cinnamon
- 1 cup fresh blueberries

- Add the cinnamon and then mix well in the fridge.
- Cook for at least 8 minutes until the milk is absorbed.
- Add the blue and light blue and then mix for a further 30 seconds.
- Serve.

13) Amaranth porridge

Preparation time: 5 minutes. **Cooking time:** 30 minutes. **Portions: 2**

Ingredients:
- 2 cups coconut milk
- 2 cups alkaline water
- 1 cup of administrator

Directions:
- In a bowl, mix the milk with the water and then boil the milk.

Ingredients:
- 2 tbsps. Coconut oil
- 1 tbsp. land cinnamon

- You put in the amaranth and then reduce the heat and make milk.

LUNCH

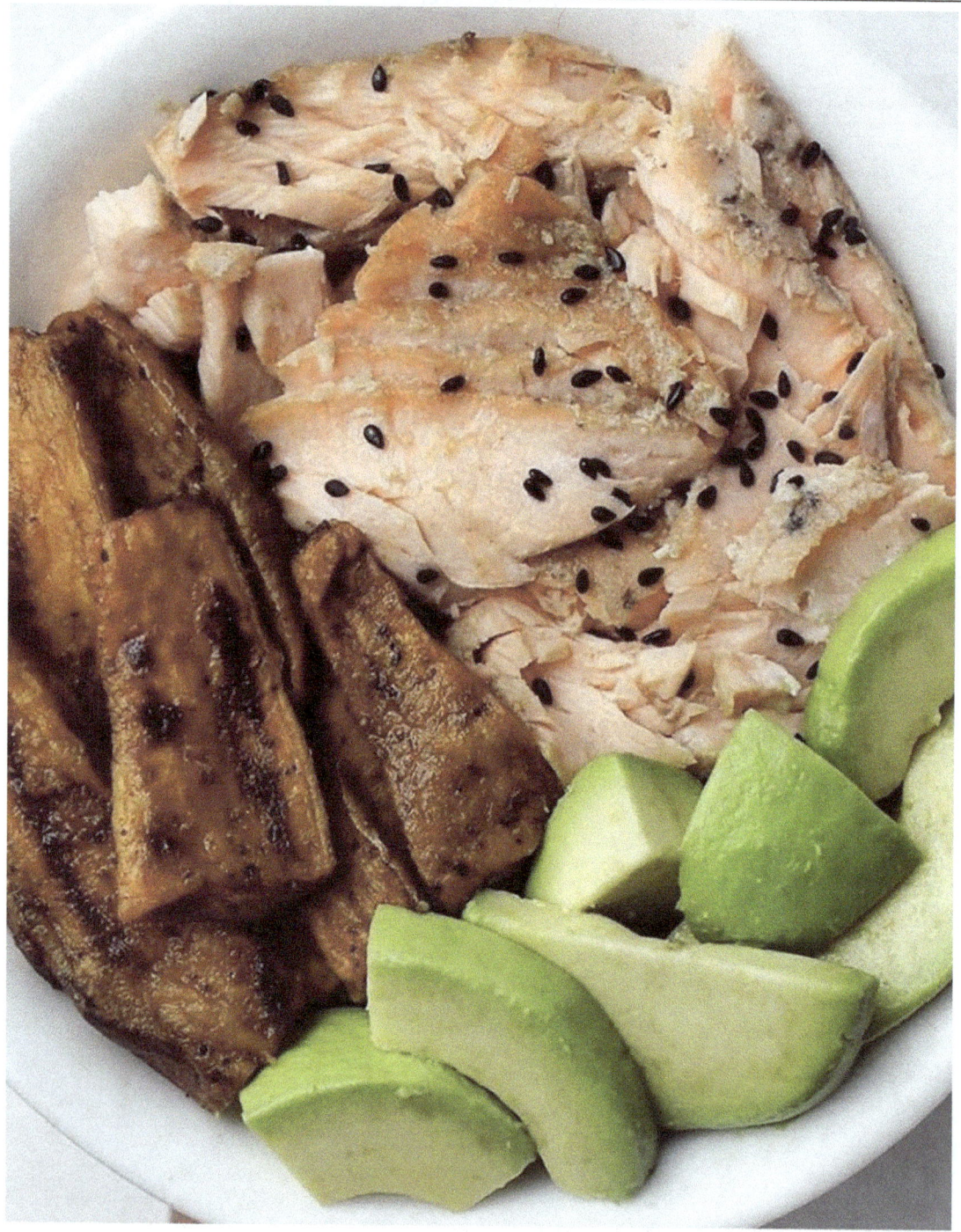

14) Wakame and pepper salad

Preparation time: 15 minutes **Cooking time:** 0 minutes **Portions:** 2

Ingredients:
- 1 cup of wakame stalks
- ½ tablespoon chopped red pepper
- ½ teaspoon of onion powder
- ½ tablespoon lime juice

Ingredients:
- ½ tablespoon agave syrup
- ½ tablespoon sesame seeds
- ½ tablespoon sesame oil

Directions:
- Put the wakame stalks in a bowl, cover with water, let them soak for 10 minutes and then drain.
- Meanwhile, prepare the dressing and for this, take a small bowl, add the lime juice, onion, agave syrup and sesame oil and then whisk until combined.
- Place the drained wakame stalks in a large dish, add the pepper, pour in the seasoning and stir until coated.
- Sprinkle the salad with sesame seeds and serve.

15) Green salad of orange and avocado

Preparation time: 5 minutes **Cooking time:** 0 minutes **Portions:** 2

Ingredients:
- 1 orange, peeled, sliced
- 4 cups of vegetables
- ½ avocado, peeled, pitted and diced
- 2 tablespoons chopped red onion
- ½ cup of coriander

Ingredients:
- ¼ teaspoon of salt
- ¼ cup of olive oil
- 2 tablespoons of lime juice
- 2 tablespoons of orange juice

Directions:
- Prepare the dressing and for this, place the coriander in a food processor, pour in the orange juice, lime juice and oil, add the salt and then pulse until combined.
- Pour the dressing into a jar. Add the remaining ingredients, stir until coated and add to a salad bowl or serve in the jar.

16) Green salad with cucumbers and mushrooms

Preparation time: 5 minutes **Cooking time:** 0 minutes **Portions:** 2

Ingredients:
- ½ medium-sized cucumber, seedless, chopped
- 6 lettuce leaves, broken into pieces
- 4 mushrooms, chopped
- 6 cherry tomatoes, chopped

Ingredients:
- 10 olives
- ½ of a lime, squeezed
- 1 teaspoon of olive oil
- ¼ teaspoon of salt
- Serve immediately.

Directions:
- Take a medium salad bowl, put all the ingredients in it and then toss until mixed.

17) Chickpea, vegetable and fonio salad

Preparation time: 10 minutes **Cooking time:** 5 minutes **Portions:** 2

Ingredients:
- ½ cup of cooked chickpeas
- ¼ cup chopped cucumber
- ½ cup crushed red pepper
- ½ cup cherry tomatoes, halved
- ½ cup of fonio

Ingredients:
- ⅓ teaspoon of salt
- 1 tablespoon of grape oil
- ⅛ teaspoon of cayenne pepper
- 1 key file, squeezed
- 1 cup of spring water

Directions:
- Take a medium saucepan, place it over high heat, pour in the water and bring it to the boil.
- Add the fonio, lower the heat, cook for 1 minute and then remove the pan from the heat.
- Cover the pot with its lid, let the fonio stand for 5 minutes, mash it with a fork and then leave it to cool for 15 minutes.
- Take a salad bowl, put in the lime juice and oil and then stir in the salt and cayenne pepper until combined.
- Add the remaining ingredients, including the fonio, stir until combined, then serve.

18) Avocado and chickpea salad

Preparation time: 10 minutes **Cooking time**: 20 minutes **Portions**: 2

Ingredients:
- ½ cucumber, seedless, sliced
- 2 avocados, peeled, pitted and diced
- 1 medium white onion, peeled, diced
- 2 cups of cooked chickpeas
- ¼ cup chopped coriander
- 1 teaspoon of onion powder

Directions:
- Turn on the oven, then set it to 425°F (220°C) and let it preheat.
- Meanwhile, take a baking tray, place the chickpeas on it, season with salt, onion powder and pepper, drizzle with oil and then toss until combined.

Ingredients:
- ½ teaspoon of cayenne pepper
- 1 teaspoon sea salt
- 2 tablespoons hemp seeds, shelled
- 1 key file, squeezed
- 1 tablespoon olive oil

- Cook the chickpeas for 20 minutes or until golden and crispy, then leave to cool for 10 minutes.
- Transfer the chickpeas to a bowl, add the remaining ingredients and stir until combined. Serve immediately.

19) Amaranth, cucumber and chickpea salad

Preparation time: 5 minutes **Cooking time**: 10 minutes **Portions**: 2

Ingredients:
- 1 small white onion, peeled, chopped
- 1 cup cooked amaranth
- ½ cucumber, seedless, chopped
- 1 cup of cooked chickpeas

Directions:
- Take a small bowl, put in the lime juice, add salt and stir until combined.

Ingredients:
- ½ of a medium red pepper, chopped
- ⅓ teaspoon of sea salt
- ⅛ teaspoon of cayenne pepper
- 2 tablespoons of lime juice

- Place the remaining ingredients in a salad bowl, drizzle with the lime juice mixture, mix and serve.

20) Avocado and rocket salad with citrus fruits

Preparation time: 5 minutes **Cooking time**: 0 minutes **Portions**: 2

Ingredients:
- 4 slices of onion
- ½ avocado, peeled, pitted and sliced
- 4 ounces (113 g) arugula
- 1 orange, peeled and sliced
- 1 teaspoon agave syrup

Ingredients:
- ⅛ teaspoon of salt
- ⅛ teaspoon of cayenne pepper
- 2 tablespoons of lime juice
- 2 tablespoons of olive oil

Directions:
- Distribute avocado, oranges, onion and rocket between two plates.
- Mix together the oil, salt, cayenne pepper, agave syrup and lime juice in a small bowl and then stir until combined.
- Pour the dressing over the salad and then serve.

21) Avocado salad and spelt noodles

Preparation time: 10 minutes **Cooking time**: 0 minutes **Portions**: 2

Ingredients:
- ½ cup avocado, peeled, pitted and chopped
- ½ cup of basil leaves
- ½ cup cherry tomatoes
- 2 cups of cooked spelt noodles

Ingredients:
- 1 teaspoon agave syrup
- 1 tablespoon lime juice
- 2 tablespoons of olive oil

Directions:
- Take a large bowl, put the pasta in it, add the tomato, avocado and basil and then mix until everything is combined.
- Take a small bowl, add the agave syrup and salt, pour in the lime juice and olive oil, and then whisk until combined.
- Pour the lime juice mixture over the pasta, stir until combined and then serve.

388 | fat: 16.5g | protein: 9.3g | carbohydrate: 54.2g | fibre: 8.5g

22) Lettuce salad with basil

Preparation time: 10 minutes **Cooking time**: 10 minutes **Portions**: 2

Ingredients:
- 2 small heads of romaine lettuce, cut in half
- 1 tablespoon chopped basil
- 1 tablespoon chopped red onion
- ¼ teaspoon of onion powder
- ½ tablespoon agave syrup

Ingredients:
- ½ teaspoon of salt
- ¼ teaspoon cayenne pepper
- 2 tablespoons of olive oil
- 1 tablespoon lime juice

Directions:
- Take a large frying pan, put it over a medium heat and when it is hot, place the heads of lettuce in it, cut side down, and then cook them for 4 to 5 minutes per side until they are golden brown on both sides.
- When finished, transfer the heads of lettuce to a plate and leave to cool for 5 minutes.
- In the meantime, prepare the dressing and for this, place the remaining ingredients in a small bowl and then mix until combined.
- Pour the dressing over the heads of lettuce and then serve.

23) Cabbage and sprout salad

Preparation time: 5 minutes **Cooking time**: 0 minutes **Portions**: 2

Ingredients:
- 2 cups of kale leaves
- 1 cup of sprouts
- 1 cup cherry tomatoes
- ½ avocado, peeled, pitted and diced

Ingredients:
- 1 key file, squeezed
- 1 teaspoon agave syrup
- ½ tablespoon olive oil
- ⅛ teaspoon of cayenne pepper

Directions:
- Take a small bowl, put the lime juice in it, add the oil and agave syrup and then stir until combined.
- Take a salad bowl, put the remaining ingredients in, drizzle with the lime juice mixture and then toss until mixed.
- Serve immediately.

24) Watercress and cucumber salad

Preparation time: 5 minutes   **Cooking time:** 0 minutes   **Portions:** 2

Ingredients:
- 2 cups of torn cress
- ½ sliced cucumber
- 1 tablespoon lime juice

Directions:
- Pour the lime juice and olive oil into a salad bowl and mix well to combine.
- Slice the cucumber and add it to the bowl.

Ingredients:
- 2 tablespoons of olive oil
- Pure sea salt, to taste
- Cayenne powder, to taste
- Tear up the watercress and add it to the bowl.
- Sprinkle with cayenne powder and pure sea salt according to your taste.
- Mix thoroughly.
- Serve immediately.

25) Watercress and orange salad

Preparation time: 10 minutes   **Cooking time:** 0 minutes   **Portions:** 2

Ingredients:
- 4 cups of torn cress
- 1 sliced avocado
- 2 thinly sliced red onions
- 1 Seville orange, chopped
- 2 tablespoons of lime juice

Directions:
- Prepare the avocado. cut it in half, peel it, remove the seeds and slice it.
- Peel the Seville orange and cut it into medium cubes.
- Remove the skin from the red onions and slice them thinly.

Ingredients:
- 2 teaspoons agave syrup
- ⅛ teaspoon of pure sea salt
- Cayenne powder, to taste
- 2 tablespoons of olive oil
- Put the onions, avocado, oranges and watercress in a salad bowl.
- Combine the olive oil, cayenne powder, pure sea salt, lime juice and agave syrup in a separate bowl, mix well.
- Pour the dressing over the top of the salad.
- Serve immediately.

26) Mushroom and olive salad

Preparation time: 10 minutes   **Cooking time:** 0 minutes   **Portions:** 2

Ingredients:
- 5 mushrooms cut in half
- 6 halved cherry (plum) tomatoes
- 6 lettuce leaves, rinsed
- 10 olives

Directions:
- Cut the rinsed lettuce leaves into medium pieces and place them in a medium salad bowl.
- Add the mushroom halves, chopped cucumber, olives and cherry tomato halves to the bowl.

Ingredients:
- ½ chopped cucumber
- Juice of ½ lime
- 1 teaspoon of olive oil
- Pure sea salt, to taste
- Stir well.
- Pour olive oil and lime juice over the salad.
- Add pure sea salt to taste. stir until well combined.
- Serve immediately.

27) Asparagus salad with cashew sauce

Preparation time: 10 minutes **Cooking time:** 5 minutes **Portions:** 1-2

Ingredients:

For the salad:
- 1 teaspoon avocado oil
- 24 asparagus stalks, diced
- ½ cup diced onion
- 3 cloves of garlic, crushed
- ½ teaspoon of sea salt
- ¼ teaspoon freshly ground black pepper

Ingredients:

For the dressing:
- ½ cup of raw cashews
- ½ cup of water
- 2 tablespoons freshly squeezed lemon juice
- ¼ teaspoon of sea salt
- ⅛ teaspoon of freshly ground black pepper

For mounting:
- 2 cups of mixed salad
- To prepare the asparagus mixture

Directions:

- To prepare the asparagus mixture
- In a large frying pan over medium heat, heat the avocado oil. Add the asparagus, onion, garlic, salt and pepper and fry for 5-7 minutes, or until the onion is soft.
- Prepare the dressing
- In a high-speed blender, blend together half of the asparagus mixture with the cashews, water, lemon juice, salt and pepper until smooth.
- To assemble the salad
- Arrange the salad mix on 1 large or 2 small plates. Add the rest of the asparagus, drizzle with the dressing and enjoy.

28) Sweet potato salad with jalapeno sauce

Preparation time: 10 minutes **Cooking time:** 25 minutes **Portions:** 1-2

Ingredients:

For sweet potatoes:
- 3 medium sweet potatoes, peeled and diced
- 2 tablespoons of avocado oil
- 2 cloves of garlic, crushed
- 1 teaspoon ground paprika
- ½ teaspoon of sea salt

For Jalapeño Dressing:
- 1 cup of water
- 1 cup raw cashews

Ingredients:

- ¼ cup of fresh coriander leaves
- ½ to 1 jalapeño
- 2 tablespoons freshly squeezed lime juice
- ½ teaspoon of sea salt

For mounting:
- 2 cups of mixed salad

Directions:

- Preheat the oven to 350ºF (180ºC). Line a baking tray with baking paper.
- To prepare the sweet potatoes
- In a medium bowl, mix the sweet potatoes, avocado oil, garlic, paprika and salt.
- Spread the sweet potato cubes evenly over the prepared baking tray and bake for 25 minutes, or until soft.
- To prepare the jalapeño dressing
- Meanwhile, in a high-speed blender, blend together the water, cashews, cilantro, jalapeño, lime juice and salt until smooth.
- To assemble
- Arrange the salad mix on 1 large or 2 small plates. Add the hot sweet potatoes, drizzle with the dressing and enjoy.

29) Green pineapple salad

Preparation time: 10 minutes	**Cooking time:** 0 minutes	**Portions: 1-2**

Ingredients:
- For the lime vinaigrette:
- ¼ cup avocado oil
- ¼ cup of water
- 2 tablespoons freshly squeezed lime juice
- ½ cup chopped shallots
- ½ cup of chopped fresh coriander
- 2 garlic cloves
- ½ teaspoon of sea salt

Directions:
- To prepare the vinaigrette
- In a blender, blend together the avocado oil, water, lime juice, onion, cilantro, garlic and salt until well combined. Adjust the seasonings as necessary.

Ingredients:
- For mounting:
- 2 to 3 cups of mixed salad
- ½ cup of diced pineapple
- 1 cup chopped purple cabbage
- Dulse flakes, for garnish (optional)

- To assemble the salad
- Arrange the salad mix on 1 large or 2 small plates. Add the pineapple, purple cabbage and dulse flakes (if using); drizzle with the dressing and serve.

30) Sweet Peach Tahini Salad

Preparation time: 10 minutes	**Cooking time:** 0 minutes	**Portions: 1-2**

Ingredients:
- 4 tablespoons of tahini
- 3 to 4 tablespoons brown rice syrup
- ¼ cup of water
- 1 teaspoon freshly squeezed lemon juice
- Pinch of sea salt
- 1 peach, pitted and cut into cubes

Directions:
- In a small bowl, whisk together the tahini, brown rice syrup, water, lemon juice and salt until well combined. Adjust seasonings as needed.

Ingredients:
- ¼ cup diced red pepper
- 1 tablespoon fresh coriander, chopped
- 1 tablespoon diced red onion
- ½ jalapeño, diced
- 2 to 3 cups of mixed salad

- In another small bowl, put together the peach, pepper, cilantro, onion and jalapeño.
- Arrange the salad mix on 1 large or 2 small plates. Add the dressing, drizzle with the dressing and enjoy.

31) Pasta salad with red lentils and vegetables

Preparation time: 15 minutes	**Cooking time:** 15 minutes	**Portions: 2-4**

Ingredients:
- 2 cups of red lentil paste
- ¼ cup avocado oil
- 2 tablespoons apple cider vinegar
- 1 tablespoon freshly squeezed lemon juice
- 1 teaspoon dried oregano
- 2 pinches of sea salt
- 2 pinches of freshly ground black pepper

Directions:
- Cook the pasta according to the package directions.
- While the pasta is cooking, in a small bowl, whisk together the avocado oil, vinegar, lemon juice, oregano, salt and pepper until well combined. Adjust seasonings as needed.

Ingredients:
- 1 tablespoon avocado oil
- 6 asparagus stalks, diced
- 1 cup of diced orange pepper
- ⅓ cup of diced red onion
- ½ courgette, sliced
- ½ summer squash, sliced
- 2 cloves of garlic, crushed

- In a frying pan over medium-high heat, heat the avocado oil. Add the asparagus, pepper, onion, courgette, pumpkin and garlic and fry for 2 to 3 minutes, or just until soft.
- In a large bowl, mix the cooked pasta, vegetables and seasoning until well combined. Transfer to 2 large or 4 small plates and enjoy.

32) Fennel and carrot salad

Preparation time: 5 minutes **Cooking time**: 0 minutes **Portions: 4**

Ingredients:
- 1 cup chopped fennel
- 1 cup of shredded carrots
- ¼ cup sliced almonds
- 3 tablespoons of sultanas
- 1 tablespoon avocado oil

Ingredients:
- 1 tablespoon freshly squeezed lemon juice
- 1 teaspoon apple cider vinegar
- 1 teaspoon Dijon or yellow mustard
- 1 teaspoon of finely grated fresh ginger or 1 cube of frozen ginger

Directions:
- In a medium bowl, mix fennel, carrots, almonds and sultanas; set aside.
- In a small bowl, whisk together the oil, lemon juice, vinegar, mustard and ginger until well combined.
- Pour the dressing over the salad and toss until evenly coated.
- Serve cold or at room temperature. Store leftovers in an airtight container in the fridge for up to 1 week.

33) Tofu and watermelon salad

Preparation time: 10 minutes **Cooking time:** 0 minutes **Portions: 4**

Ingredients:
- 2 tablespoons freshly squeezed lemon juice
- 2 tablespoons of avocado oil
- 1 teaspoon dried oregano
- ½ teaspoon dried thyme
- ¼ teaspoon of garlic powder
- ¼ teaspoon of sea salt

Ingredients:
- 8 ounces (227 g) solid tofu, cubed
- ¼ cup balsamic vinegar
- 8 dates, pitted
- 4 cups of crunchy leafy vegetables
- 1 cup of diced watermelon
- ¼ cup fresh basil, chopped

Directions:
- In a small bowl, combine the lemon juice, oil, oregano, thyme, garlic powder and salt. Add the tofu and let it absorb the flavours while you prepare the salad.
- In a high-speed blender, combine the vinegar and dates and blend until smooth.
- In each of 4 salad bowls, place 1 cup of leafy greens. Add ¼ cup of watermelon to each.
- Using a slotted spoon, cover each bowl with 2 tablespoons of vegan feta (store the remaining vegan feta in an airtight container in the fridge for up to 5 days).
- Garnish evenly with the basil. Pour a spoonful of balsamic mixture over each salad and serve.

34) Spinach and strawberry salad with lemon vinaigrette

Preparation time: 5 minutes **Cooking time:** 0 minutes **Portions: 4**

Ingredients:
For the lemon vinaigrette
- 3 tablespoons avocado oil
- Juice of 1 small lemon
- 1 teaspoon Dijon or yellow mustard
- ¼ teaspoon ground turmeric
- ⅛ teaspoon of sea salt

Ingredients:
- 1 teaspoon maple syrup (optional)
For the salad:
- 4 cups baby spinach
- 1 cup of strawberries cut in half
- ¼ cup sliced almonds

Directions:
- To make the lemon vinaigrette
- In a small bowl, whisk together the oil, lemon juice, mustard, turmeric and salt until well combined. Add the maple syrup (if using) and mix well.
- To make the salad
- In a large bowl, mix the spinach, strawberries and almonds.
- Pour the dressing over the salad and toss gently. Serve immediately. Or, if you plan to serve later, store the unseasoned salad and dressing in separate airtight containers in the refrigerator and add the dressing to the salad when you are ready to serve.

35) Rainbow salad with citrus mango dressing

Preparation time: 5 minutes   **Cooking time:** 0 minutes   **Portions:** 4

Ingredients:

For the citrus mango salsa:
- 2 cups of chopped mango
- 1 cup chopped fennel
- ⅓ cup of chopped shallot
- ¼ cup fresh basil, chopped
- 3 tablespoons freshly squeezed lemon juice
- ¼ teaspoon of sea salt

Directions:
- To make the citrus mango salsa
- In a medium bowl, combine the mango, fennel, shallot, basil, lemon juice and salt and mix well. For best results, cover and refrigerate for several hours or up to overnight to allow the flavours to meld.

Ingredients:

For the rainbow salad:
- 1 (15-ounce / 425-g) can low-sodium chickpeas, drained (reserved liquid) and rinsed
- ½ cup chopped pepper
- 1 teaspoon chopped fresh coriander, for garnish

- To make the rainbow salad
- In a large bowl, combine the chickpeas, pepper and ¼ cup of the sauce. (Store the remaining sauce in an airtight container in the refrigerator for 5-7 days).
- Garnish the salad with coriander and serve.

36) Roasted cabbage and beetroot salad

Preparation time: 10 minutes   **Cooking time:** 20 minutes   **Portions:** 1-2

Ingredients:
- 4 small beets, peeled and diced
- 1 teaspoon avocado oil
- ¼ teaspoon dried rosemary
- ⅛ teaspoon of garlic powder
- Pinch of sea salt
- Pinch of freshly ground black pepper
- 2 cups of chopped kale

Directions:
- Preheat the oven to 400ºF (205ºC). Line a baking tray with baking paper.
- In a small bowl, mix the beetroot with the avocado oil to coat. Sprinkle with the rosemary, garlic powder, salt and pepper and toss to coat. Transfer the beets to the prepared baking dish and roast for 15-20 minutes, or until slightly crispy.

Ingredients:
- ⅛ teaspoon of sea salt
- 2 tablespoons of avocado oil
- 1 tablespoon freshly squeezed lemon juice
- 1 tablespoon brown rice syrup
- 1 clove of garlic, crushed
- Pinch of sea salt
- Pinch of freshly ground black pepper

- Meanwhile, in a medium bowl, sprinkle the cabbage with the salt, and gently massage the cabbage with your hands, crushing it until soft and slightly mushy, about 3 minutes. Transfer to a serving dish.
- In a small bowl, whisk together the avocado oil, lemon juice, brown rice syrup, garlic, salt and pepper until well combined.
- Add the beetroot to the bowl with the cabbage and drizzle with the dressing. Transfer to 1 large or 2 small plates and enjoy.

37) Spelt pasta with avocado

Preparation time: 20 minutes   **Cooking time:** 0 minutes   **Portions:** 4

Ingredients:
- 4 cups of cooked spelt pasta
- 1 medium avocado, diced
- 2 cups of halved cherry tomatoes
- 1 fresh basil, chopped

Directions:
- Place the cooked pasta in a large bowl.
- Add the diced avocado, halved cherry tomatoes and chopped basil to the bowl.
- Mix all ingredients together until well combined.

Ingredients:
- 1 teaspoon agave syrup
- 1 tablespoon lime juice
- ¼ cup of olive oil

- Whisk the agave syrup, olive oil, pure sea salt and lime juice in a separate bowl.
- Pour it over the dough and stir until well combined.
- Serve immediately.

38) Lettuce and mushroom burger with basil

Preparation time: 15 minutes **Cooking time:** 20 minutes **Portions: 2**

Ingredients:
- 2 cups portobello mushroom caps
- 1 sliced avocado
- 1 sliced plum tomato
- 1 cup of torn lettuce
- 1 cup of purslane

Ingredients:
- ½ teaspoon of cayenne
- 1 teaspoon of oregano
- 2 teaspoons of basil
- 3 tablespoons of olive oil

Directions:
- Preheat oven to 425°F (220°C).
- Remove the mushroom stems and cut a ½ inch slice from the top slice, as if slicing a sandwich.
- Mix the onion powder, cayenne, oregano, olive oil and basil well in a medium bowl.
- Cover a baking tray with aluminium foil and brush with grapeseed oil to prevent sticking.
- Place the mushroom caps on a baking tray and brush with the prepared marinade. Marinate for 10 minutes before baking.
- Bake for 10 minutes until golden brown and then turn upside down. Continue baking for a further 10 minutes.
- Spread the mushroom cap on a serving plate. This will serve as a base for the mushroom burger. On top of it, make a layer of sliced avocado, tomatoes, lettuce and purslane.
- Cover the burger with another mushroom cap. Repeat steps 7 and 8 with the remaining mushrooms and vegetables.
- Serve and enjoy.

39) Zoodles with tomato sauce and avocado

Preparation time: 10 minutes **Cooking time:** 15-20 minutes **Portions: 3**

Ingredients:
- 3 medium-sized courgettes
- 1½ cups of cherry tomatoes
- 1 avocado
- 2 sliced green onions
- ⅓ cup of fresh parsley
- 1 garlic clove

Ingredients:
- 3 tablespoons of olive oil
- Juice of 1 key lemon
- 1 tablespoon of spring water
- Pure sea salt, to taste
- Cayenne, to taste

Directions:
- Preheat the oven to 400°F (205°C).
- Cover a baking tray with a piece of baking paper.
- Place the cherry tomatoes on a covered baking tray. Drizzle with 1 tablespoon of olive oil and season with pure sea salt and cayenne.
- Cook the tomatoes for about 15-20 minutes until they start to split.
- Add the avocado quarters, torn parsley leaves, sliced green onions, garlic, spring water, key lime juice and ½ teaspoon pure sea salt to a food processor.
- Blend until a creamy consistency is achieved. If the sauce is too thick, add more spring water.
- Cut the ends off the courgettes. Using a spiraliser, make courgette noodles.
- Mix the courgette noodles with the prepared avocado sauce.
- Divide between 3 small bowls and serve with cherry tomatoes.
- Enjoy your zoodles with sauce!

40) Mushroom and pepper fajitas

Preparation time: 10 minutes **Cooking time:** 10 minutes **Portions: 3**

Ingredients:
- 6 tortillas
- 3 large portobello mushrooms
- 1 onion
- 2 peppers
- 1 teaspoon onion powder

Ingredients:
- 1 teaspoon habanero pepper
- ⅛ teaspoon of cayenne powder
- Juice of ½ key lime
- 1 tablespoon grape seed oil

Directions:
- Rinse the portobello mushrooms and remove the stalks. Cut into ⅓-inch slices.
- Cut the onion and peppers into thin slices.
- Add the grapeseed oil to a large frying pan and heat over a medium heat. Add the sliced onions and peppers and cook for 2 minutes.
- Place the sliced mushrooms and seasoning in the pan. Cook for 7-8 minutes, stirring occasionally. Remove from the heat.
- Take a small frying pan, place the tortillas on it and heat for 30-60 seconds on each side.
- Place the filling mixture in the centre of the tortillas and pour the lime juice over the vegetables.
- Serve and enjoy.

41) Chickpea and mushroom sausages

Preparation time: 15 minutes **Cooking time:** 5 minutes **Portions: 8-10**

Ingredients:
- 2 cups of cooked chickpeas
- 1 quart of Roma tomato
- 1 cup of quartered mushrooms
- ½ cup chopped onion
- ½ cup of chickpea flour
- 1 tablespoon onion powder
- 1 teaspoon of ground sage
- 1 teaspoon of basil

Ingredients:
- 1 teaspoon of oregano
- 1 teaspoon of dill
- ½ teaspoon of ground cloves
- 1 teaspoon pure sea salt
- ½ teaspoon of cayenne powder
- 2 tablespoons of grape seed oil

Directions:
- Put all the ingredients, except the chickpea flour and grape seed oil, into a food processor.
- Blend for 15 seconds.
- Add the chickpea flour to the mixture and blend for a further 30 seconds until well combined.
- Place the mixture in a piping bag and cut a small piece from the bottom corner.
- Add the grapeseed oil to a frying pan and heat over high heat.
- Reduce to a medium heat. Squeeze the prepared mixture into the pan to form sausages.
- Cook them for about 3 to 4 minutes on all sides. Turn carefully to prevent them from falling apart.
- Serve and enjoy.

42) Mushroom and kale ravioli

Preparation time: 25 minutes **Cooking time:** 10 minutes **Portions: 5**

Ingredients:
Filling:
- 1 cup of chickpea flour
- 1 quart of Roma tomato
- 2 cups of quartered mushrooms
- 1 cup of chopped cabbage
- ⅓ cup of diced onions
- 1 cup diced green and red peppers
- 1 tablespoon onion powder
- 1 teaspoon of ginger
- 2 teaspoons of oregano
- 2 teaspoons of dill
- 2 teaspoons of basil
- 2 teaspoons of thyme
- 1 teaspoon pure sea salt
- ½ teaspoon of cayenne

Ingredients:
Dough:
- ½ cup of chickpea flour
- 1½ cups of spelt flour
- ½ teaspoon of oregano
- ½ teaspoon of basil
- 1 teaspoon pure sea salt
- ¾ cup of spring water

Cheese:
- ½ cup of soaked Brazil nuts (overnight or for at least 3 hours)
- 2 teaspoons of onion powder
- ½ teaspoon of oregano
- 1 teaspoon pure sea salt
- ½ teaspoon of cayenne powder
- ½ cup of spring water

Directions:
- Blend all the filling ingredients, except the chickpea flour, in a food processor for 30-40 seconds.
- Add the chickpea flour to the mixture and blend until well combined.
- Add the grapeseed oil to a frying pan and heat over high heat.
- Reduce to a medium heat. Distribute the ravioli filling in the pan and cook for 3 to 4 minutes on all sides.
- Break up the filling and cook for a further 3 minutes, then transfer to a medium bowl.
- Add all the ingredients for the cheese to the food processor and blend until the consistency is creamy. If it is too thick, add a little spring water.
- Mix the filling with the cheese mixture in the bowl.
- Place all the dry ingredients for the dough in the food processor and blend for 10-20 seconds. Slowly add the spring water while blending, until the dough can be shaped into a ball.
- Spread the flour on the work surface. Take ¼ of the dough and roll it out into a thin sheet.
- Place rounded teaspoons of filling and cheese 1 inch apart on one side of the dough. Fold the dough and press together around the filling to seal. Cut into individual ravioli with a pastry cutter or knife.
- Repeat steps 9 and 10 with the remaining dough and filling.
- Bring a pot of spring water to the boil. add a little pure sea salt and grapeseed oil, then cook the ravioli for about 4-6 minutes.
- Filter and serve.

43) Lettuce wrap and courgette hummus

Preparation time: 10 minutes **Cooking time:** 8 minutes **Portions:** 2

Ingredients:
- ½ cup iceberg lettuce
- 1 courgette, sliced
- 2 cherry tomatoes, sliced
- 2 spelt flour tortillas

Directions:
- Take a grill pan, grease it with oil and preheat it over medium-high heat.
- Meanwhile, place the courgette slices in a large bowl, sprinkle with salt and cayenne pepper, drizzle with oil and then toss until coated.
- Place the courgette slices on the grill pan and then cook for 2 to 3 minutes per side until grill marks develop.

Ingredients:
- 4 tablespoons of homemade hummus
- ¼ teaspoon of salt
- ⅛ teaspoon of cayenne pepper
- 1 tablespoon of grape oil
- Assemble the tortillas and for this, heat the tortilla on the grill pan until grill marks develop and spread 2 tablespoons of hummus on each tortilla.
- Spread the grilled courgette slices on the tortillas, cover with lettuce and tomato slices, then wrap tightly.
- Serve immediately.

44) Apple and pumpkin burger by Butternut

Preparation time: 10 minutes **Cooking time:** 1 hour **Portions:** 2

Ingredients:
- ¾ cup diced pumpkin
- ½ cup diced apples
- 1 cup cooked wild rice
- ¼ cup chopped shallots
- ½ tablespoon of thyme

Directions:
- Turn on the oven, then set it to 400°F (205°C) and let it preheat.
- In the meantime, take a biscuit tin, line it with a sheet of parchment, spread the pumpkin pieces on it and then sprinkle with ⅛ teaspoon of salt.
- Cook the pumpkin for 15 minutes, then add the shallot and apple, sprinkle with the remaining salt and cook for 20-30 minutes until cooked through.
- When finished, leave the vegetable mixture to cool for 15 minutes, transfer it to a food processor, add the thyme and then pulse until the mixture is chunky.

Ingredients:
- ¼ teaspoon of sea salt, divided by
- 1 tablespoon unsalted pumpkin seeds
- 1 tablespoon of grape oil
- 2 spelt burgers, halved, toasted

- Add the pumpkin seeds and cooked wild rice, pulse until combined, then tip the mixture into a bowl.
- Taste the mixture to adjust it and then shape it into two meatballs.
- Take a frying pan, place it over a medium heat, add the oil and when it is hot, place the meatballs in it and cook for 5 to 7 minutes per side until golden brown.
- Place the patties in hamburger buns and then serve.

45) Cabbage and avocado

Preparation time: 5 minutes **Cooking time:** 0 minutes **Portions:** 2

Ingredients:
- 1 bundle of cabbage, cut into thin strips
- 1 small white onion, peeled, chopped
- 12 cherry tomatoes, chopped

Directions:
- Take a large bowl, place the cabbage strips in it, sprinkle with salt and then massage for 2 minutes.

Ingredients:
- 1 tablespoon salt
- 1 avocado, peeled, stoned, sliced

- Cover the bowl with plastic wrap or its lid, let it stand for a minimum of 30 minutes, and then stir in the onion and tomatoes until well combined.
- Let the salad rest for 5 minutes, add the avocado slices and then serve.

46) Courgette bacon

Preparation time: 10 minutes **Cooking time**: 20 minutes **Portions**: 2

Ingredients:
- ✓ 2 courgettes, cut into strips
- ✓ 1 tablespoon onion powder
- ✓ 1 tablespoon sea salt
- ✓ ½ teaspoon of cayenne powder
- ✓ ¼ cup of date sugar

Directions:
- ❖ Take a medium saucepan, put it over medium heat, add all the ingredients except the courgettes and the oil and then cook until the sugar has dissolved.
- ❖ Then place the courgette strips in a large bowl, pour in the casserole mixture, stir until coated, and then leave to marinate for a minimum of 1 hour.

Ingredients:
- ✓ 2 tablespoons agave syrup
- ✓ 1 teaspoon of liquid smoke
- ✓ ¼ cup of spring water
- ✓ 1 tablespoon of grape oil

- ❖ When you are ready to cook, turn on the oven, set it to 400ºF (205ºC) and let it preheat.
- ❖ Take a baking tray, line it with a sheet of parchment, grease it with oil, place the marinated courgette strips on top and then bake for 10 minutes.
- ❖ Then turn the courgettes over, continue cooking for 4 minutes and then leave to cool completely.
- ❖ Serve immediately.

47) Mushroom and pepper fritters

Preparation time: 10 minutes **Cooking time**: 10 minutes **Portions**: 2

Ingredients:
- ✓ 1 cup of chickpea flour
- ✓ 7 ounces (198 g) mushrooms, chopped
- ✓ 1 medium green pepper, core, chopped
- ✓ 1 tablespoon onion powder
- ✓ 2 medium-sized white onions, peeled, chopped
- ✓ 1 teaspoon sea salt

Directions:
- ❖ Take a large bowl, put all the vegetables, add all the seasonings, basil and oregano, mix until combined and then leave the mixture to stand for 5 minutes.
- ❖ Add the chickpea flour, stir until combined and then stir in the water until well combined and smooth.

Ingredients:
- ✓ 1 tablespoon oregano
- ✓ ⅛ teaspoon of cayenne pepper
- ✓ 1 tablespoon of grape oil
- ✓ 1 tablespoon basil leaves, chopped
- ✓ ½ cup of spring water

- ❖ Take a large frying pan, place it over medium heat, add the oil and, when hot, pour the vegetable mixture into portions, press each portion down, and then cook for 3 to 4 minutes per side until cooked and golden brown.
- ❖ Serve immediately.

48) Chickpea, pepper and mushroom curry

Preparation time: 5 minutes **Cooking time**: 12 minutes **Portions**: 2

Ingredients:
- ✓ 1 cup of cooked chickpeas
- ✓ 1 small white onion, peeled, diced
- ✓ ½ of a medium green pepper, core, chopped
- ✓ 1 cup diced mushrooms

Directions:
- ❖ Take a medium-sized frying pan, place it over medium heat, add the oil and when it is hot, add the onion, tomatoes and pepper and cook for 2 minutes.

Ingredients:
- ✓ 8 cherry tomatoes, chopped
- ✓ ½ teaspoon of salt
- ✓ ¼ teaspoon cayenne pepper
- ✓ 1 teaspoon of grape oil

- ❖ Add the chickpeas and mushrooms, season with and cayenne pepper, stir until combined, and lower the heat to medium-low and then simmer for 10 minutes until cooked through, covering the pan with its lid.
- ❖ Serve immediately.

49) Spelt noodles with peppers and mushrooms

Preparation time: 5 minutes **Cooking time**: 10 minutes **Portions**: 2

Ingredients:
- 2 cups of cooked spelt noodles
- ½ of a medium green pepper, cored, cut into slices
- ½ of a medium-sized red pepper, cored, sliced
- 1 medium white onion, with core, sliced
- ½ cup of sliced mushrooms

Directions:
- Take a large frying pan, put it on a medium heat, add the oil and when it is hot, add all the vegetables and cook for 3-5 minutes until tender and crispy.

Ingredients:
- ⅔ teaspoon of salt
- ¼ teaspoon of onion powder
- ⅓ teaspoon of cayenne pepper
- 1 key lime, squeezed
- 1 tablespoon sesame oil
- Add all the spices, sprinkle with the lime juice, stir until combined, then cook for 1 minute.
- Add the noodles, stir until well mixed and then cook for 2 to 3 minutes until hot.
- Serve immediately.

50) Okra and tomato curry

Preparation time: 5 minutes **Cooking time**: 10 minutes **Portions**: 2

Ingredients:
- 1½ cups okra
- 8 cherry tomatoes, chopped
- 1 medium onion, peeled, sliced
- ¾ cup of home-made vegetable broth
- 6 teaspoons of spice mixture

Directions:
- Take a large frying pan, put it over medium heat, add the oil and heat, add the onion, and then cook for 5 minutes until golden brown.
- Add the spice mix, add the remaining ingredients to the pan except the okra, stir until combined, and then bring the mixture to a simmer.

Ingredients:
- ¼ teaspoon of salt
- ½ tablespoon of grape oil
- ¼ teaspoon cayenne pepper
- ¾ cup of tomato sauce, alkaline
- 6 tablespoons of soft coconut milk jelly
- Add the okra, stir until combined, and then cook for 10-15 minutes over medium-low heat until cooked through.
- Serve immediately.

51) Sage mushrooms in the oven

Preparation time: 10 minutes **Cooking time**: 30 minutes **Portions**: 2

Ingredients:
- 2 cups portobello mushrooms, detached
- ⅔ teaspoon of chopped onion
- ⅔ teaspoon chopped sage

Directions:
- Turn on the oven, then set it to 400°F (205°C) and let it preheat.
- Take an oven dish and then place the mushroom caps in it, cut side up.

Ingredients:
- ⅔ teaspoon of thyme
- ⅔ tablespoon of lime juice
- 2 tablespoons alkaline soy sauce
- Take a small bowl, put in the remaining ingredients, mix until combined, brush the mixture onto the inside and outside of the mushrooms, and then leave to marinate for 15 minutes.
- Cook the mushrooms for 30 minutes, turning them halfway through cooking, then serve.

52) Spelt pasta with Swiss chard

Preparation time: 5 minutes **Cooking time:** 5 minutes **Portions:** 2

Ingredients:
- 1 head of Swiss chard, cut into ½ inch pieces
- 1 cup of spelt pasta, cooked
- 2 green onions, sliced
- ¼ cup coriander

Ingredients:
- 1 key lime, squeezed, zested
- ¼ teaspoon of salt
- ¼ teaspoon cayenne pepper
- 1 tablespoon olive oil

Directions:
- Take a large frying pan, put it over a medium heat, add the oil and when it is hot, add the chard pieces and then cook for 4 minutes or more until they are wilted.
- Remove the pan from the heat, transfer the chard to a large bowl, add the remaining ingredients and then stir until combined.
- Serve immediately.

53) Baked pumpkin and apples

Preparation time: 10 minutes **Cooking time:** 35 minutes **Portions:** 2

Ingredients:
- 1½ pounds (680 g) butternut squash, peeled, seeded and cut into pieces
- 2 apples, core, cut into ½ inch pieces
- 2 tablespoons agave syrup

Ingredients:
- ½ teaspoon of sea salt
- 2 tablespoons of grape oil

Directions:
- Turn on the oven, then set it to 375°F (190°C) and let it preheat.
- Meanwhile, take a baking tray and then spread the pumpkin pieces on it.
- Take a small bowl, pour in the oil, stir in the salt and allspice until combined, then pour over the pumpkin pieces.
- Cover the pan with aluminium foil and bake for 20 minutes.
- Meanwhile, place the apple pieces in a medium bowl, drizzle with the agave syrup and stir until coated.
- When the pumpkin is cooked, discard the pan, pour the spoonful into the bowl containing the apple and then stir until combined.
- Spread the apple and pumpkin mixture evenly over the baking tray and then continue baking for 15 minutes.
- Serve immediately.

DINNER

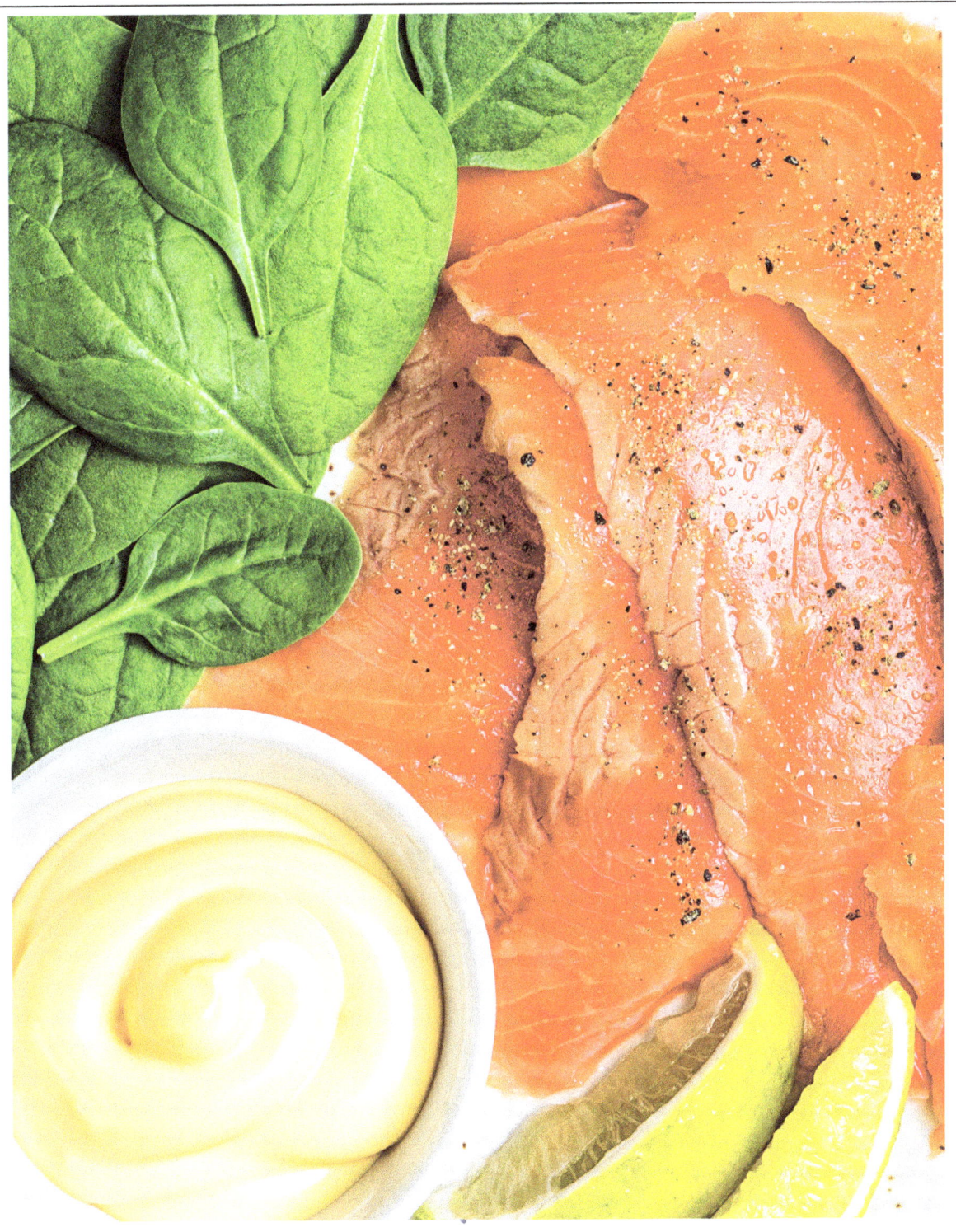

54) Vegetarian stew

Preparation time: 20 minutes   **Cooking time**: 35 minutes   **Portions**: 8

Ingredients:
- 2 tablespoons of coconut oil
- 1 large sweet onion, chopped
- 1 medium parsnip, peeled and chopped
- 3 tablespoons of homemade tomato paste
- 2 large cloves of garlic, minced
- ½ teaspoon ground cinnamon
- ½ teaspoon ground ginger
- 1 teaspoon ground cumin
- ¼ teaspoon cayenne pepper

Ingredients:
- 2 medium-sized carrots, peeled and chopped
- 2 medium purple potatoes, peeled and cut into pieces
- 2 medium sweet potatoes, peeled and cut into pieces
- 4 cups of homemade vegetable stock
- 2 cups fresh cabbage, cut and chopped
- 2 tablespoons fresh lemon juice
- Sea salt and freshly ground black pepper, to taste

Directions:
- In a large soup pot, melt the coconut oil over medium-high heat and sauté the onion for about 5 minutes.
- Add the parsnips and fry for about 3 minutes.
- Stir in the tomato paste, garlic and spices and fry for about 2 minutes.
- Stir in the carrots, potatoes, sweet potatoes and stock and bring to the boil.
- Reduce the heat to medium-low and simmer covered for about 20 minutes.
- Add the cabbage, lemon juice, salt and black pepper and simmer for about 5 minutes.
- Serve hot.

55) Quinoa and lentil stew

Preparation time: 15 minutes   **Cooking time**: 30 minutes   **Portions**: 6

Ingredients:
- 1 tablespoon of coconut oil
- 3 carrots, peeled and cut into pieces
- 3 celery stalks, chopped
- 1 yellow onion, chopped
- 4 cloves of garlic, minced
- 4 cups of tomatoes, chopped
- 1 cup of red lentils, rinsed and drained

Ingredients:
- ½ cup dried quinoa, rinsed and drained
- 1½ teaspoons of ground cumin
- 1 teaspoon of red chilli powder
- 5 cups of vegetable stock
- 2 cups fresh spinach, chopped
- Sea salt and freshly ground black pepper, to taste

Directions:
- In a large frying pan, heat the oil over medium heat and fry the celery, onion and carrot for about 4-5 minutes.
- Add the garlic and fry for about 1 minute.
- Add the remaining ingredients except the spinach and bring to the boil.
- Reduce the heat to low and simmer, covered, for about 20 minutes.
- Add the spinach and simmer for about 3-4 minutes.
- Add salt and black pepper and remove from the heat.
- Serve hot.

292; total fat 6.9 g; saturated fat 1.2 g; cholesterol 0 mg; sodium 842 mg; total carbohydrates 39.1 g; fibre 17.3 g; sugar 6.1 g; protein 19 g

56) Black bean chili

Preparation time: 15 minutes   **Cooking time**:   **Portions**: 6

Ingredients:
- 2 tablespoons of olive oil
- 1 onion, chopped
- 1 small red pepper, seeded and chopped
- 1 small green pepper, seeded and chopped
- 4 cloves of garlic, minced
- 1 teaspoon ground cumin
- 1 teaspoon cayenne pepper

Ingredients:
- 1 tablespoon of red chilli powder
- 1 medium sweet potato, peeled and cut into pieces
- 3 cups of tomatoes, finely chopped
- 4 cups of cooked, rinsed and drained black beans
- 2 cups of homemade vegetable stock
- Sea salt and freshly ground black pepper, to taste

Directions:
- In a large frying pan, heat the oil over medium-high heat and fry the onion and peppers for about 3-4 minutes.
- Add the garlic and spices and fry for about 1 minute.
- Add the sweet potato and cook for about 4-5 minutes.
- Add the remaining ingredients and bring to the boil.
- Reduce the heat to medium-low and simmer covered for about 1½-2 hours.
- Season with salt and black pepper and remove from the heat.
- Serve hot.

57) Kidney bean curry

Preparation time: 15 minutes **Cooking time:** 25 minutes **Portions: 6**

Ingredients:
- ¼ cup extra virgin olive oil
- 1 medium onion, finely chopped
- 2 cloves of garlic, minced
- 2 tablespoons fresh ginger, chopped
- 1 cup of home-made tomato puree
- 1 teaspoon ground coriander
- 1 teaspoon ground cumin
- ½ teaspoon ground turmeric

Ingredients:
- ¼ teaspoon cayenne pepper
- Sea salt and freshly ground black pepper, to taste
- 2 large plum tomatoes, finely chopped
- 3 cups of boiled red beans
- 2 cups of water
- ½ cup fresh parsley, chopped

Directions:
- In a large soup pot, heat the oil over medium heat and sauté the onion, garlic and ginger for about 4-5 minutes.
- Stir in the tomato puree and spices and cook for about 5 minutes.
- Add the tomatoes, beans and water and bring to the boil over high heat.
- Reduce the heat to medium and simmer for about 10-15 minutes or until the desired thickness.
- Serve hot and garnish with parsley.

58) Green beans in a casserole

Preparation time: 20 minutes **Cooking time:** 20 minutes **Portions: 6**

Ingredients:
- For the onion slices:
- ½ cup yellow onion, very thinly sliced
- ¼ cup almond flour
- 1/8 teaspoon of garlic powder
- Sea salt and freshly ground black pepper, to taste
- For the casserole:
- 1 pound fresh green beans, cut up
- 1 tablespoon olive oil

Ingredients:
- 8 ounces fresh cremini mushrooms, sliced
- ½ cup yellow onion, thinly sliced
- 1/8 teaspoon of garlic powder
- Sea salt and freshly ground black pepper, to taste
- 1 teaspoon fresh thyme, chopped
- ½ cup of homemade vegetable stock
- ½ cup of coconut cream

Directions:
- Preheat the oven to 350 degrees F.
- For the onion slices, place all the ingredients in a bowl and mix to coat the onion well.
- Arrange the onion slices on a large baking tray in a single layer and set aside.
- In a pot of boiling salted water, add the green beans and cook for about 5 minutes.
- Drain the green beans and transfer them to a bowl of iced water.
- Drain them well and transfer them again to a large bowl. Set them aside.
- In a large frying pan, heat the oil over medium-high heat and fry the mushrooms, onion, garlic powder, salt and black pepper for about 2-3 minutes.
- Stir in the thyme and stock and cook for about 3-5 minutes or until all the liquid is absorbed.
- Remove from the heat and transfer the mushroom mixture to the bowl with the green beans.
- Add the coconut cream and stir to combine well.
- Transfer the mixture to a 10-inch casserole dish.
- Put the casserole dish and the pan of onion slices in the oven.
- Bake for about 15-17 minutes.
- Remove the tray and foil from the oven and leave to cool for about 5 minutes before serving.
- Cover the casserole dish evenly with the crispy onion slices.
- Cut into 6 equal-sized portions and serve.

59) *Vegetarian cake*

Preparation time: 20 minutes **Cooking time**: 20 minutes **Portions**: 8

Ingredients:
For the gasket:
- ✓ 5 cups of water
- ✓ 1¼ cup of yellow maize flour

For archiving:
- ✓ 1 tablespoon extra virgin olive oil
- ✓ 1 large onion, chopped
- ✓ 1 medium red pepper, seeded and chopped

Directions:
- ❖ Preheat the oven to 375 degrees F. Lightly grease a shallow baking tray.
- ❖ In a pan, add water over medium-high heat and bring to the boil.
- ❖ Slowly add the cornflour, stirring constantly.
- ❖ Reduce the heat to low and cook covered for about 20 minutes, stirring occasionally.
- ❖ Meanwhile, prepare the filling. In a large frying pan, heat the oil over medium heat and fry the onion and pepper for about 3-4 minutes.
- ❖ Add the garlic, oregano and spices and fry for about 1 minute.
- ❖ Add the remaining ingredients and stir to combine.

Ingredients:
- ✓ 2 cloves of garlic, minced
- ✓ 1 teaspoon dried oregano, crushed
- ✓ 2 teaspoons of chilli powder
- ✓ 2 cups fresh tomatoes, chopped
- ✓ 2½ cups cooked pinto beans
- ✓ 2 cups of boiled corn kernels

- ❖ Reduce the heat to low and simmer for about 10-15 minutes, stirring occasionally.
- ❖ Remove from heat.
- ❖ Place half of the cooked cornmeal in the prepared baking tin evenly.
- ❖ Spoon the filling mixture onto the cornflour evenly.
- ❖ Place the remaining cornflour on top of the filling mixture evenly.
- ❖ Bake for 45-50 minutes or until the top is golden brown.
- ❖ Remove the cake from the oven and set aside for about 5 minutes before serving.

60) *Rice and lentil meatloaf*

Preparation time: 20 minutes **Cooking time**: 1 hour and 10 minutes **Portions**: 8

Ingredients:
- ✓ 1¾ cups plus 2 tablespoons of filtered water, divided by
- ✓ ½ cup of wild rice
- ✓ ½ cup of brown lentils
- ✓ Pinch of sea salt
- ✓ ½ teaspoon sodium-free Italian seasoning
- ✓ 1 medium yellow onion, chopped
- ✓ 1 celery stalk, chopped
- ✓ 6 cremini mushrooms, chopped

Directions:
- ❖ In a saucepan, add 1¾ cups of water, the rice, lentils, salt and Italian seasoning and bring to the boil over medium-high heat.
- ❖ Reduce the heat to low and simmer, covered, for about 45 minutes.
- ❖ Remove from the heat and set aside covered for at least 10 minutes.
- ❖ Preheat the oven to 350 degrees F.
- ❖ Using the parchment paper, line a 9x5 inch baking tin.
- ❖ In a frying pan, heat the remaining water over medium heat and fry the onion, celery, mushrooms and garlic for about 4-5 minutes.
- ❖ Remove from the heat and allow to cool slightly.

Ingredients:
- ✓ 4 cloves of garlic, minced
- ✓ ¾ cup rolled oats
- ✓ ½ cup pecans, finely chopped
- ✓ ¾ cup of home-made tomato sauce
- ✓ ½ teaspoon red pepper flakes, crushed
- ✓ 1 teaspoon fresh rosemary, chopped
- ✓ 2 teaspoons fresh thyme, chopped

- ❖ In a large bowl, add the oats, pecans, tomato sauce and fresh herbs and stir until well combined.
- ❖ Add the rice and vegetable mixture to the oat mixture and mix well.
- ❖ In a blender, add the mixture and pulse until it forms a chunky mixture.
- ❖ Transfer the mixture evenly into the prepared baking tin.
- ❖ With a piece of foil, cover the baking tray and bake for about 40 minutes.
- ❖ Uncover and cook for about 15-20 minutes more or until the top is golden brown.
- ❖ Remove from the oven and set aside for about 5-10 minutes before slicing.
- ❖ Cut into slices of the desired size and serve.

61) Asparagus risotto

Preparation time: 15 minutes **Cooking time**: 45 minutes **Portions**: 4

Ingredients:
- 15-20 fresh asparagus spears, trimmed and cut into 1½ inch pieces
- 2 tablespoons of olive oil
- 1 cup yellow onion, chopped
- 1 clove of garlic, chopped
- 1 cup Arborio rice
- 1 tablespoon fresh lemon peel, finely grated

Directions:
- Boil the water in a medium pan then add the asparagus and cook for about 3 minutes.
- Drain the asparagus and rinse under cold running water.
- Drain well and set aside.
- In a large frying pan, heat the oil over medium heat and fry the onion for about 5 minutes.
- Add the garlic and fry for about 1 minute.
- Add the rice and fry for about 2 minutes.

Ingredients:
- 2 tablespoons fresh lemon juice
- 5½ cups of hot vegetable stock
- 1 tablespoon fresh parsley, chopped
- ¼ cup of nutritional yeast
- Sea salt and freshly ground black pepper, to taste

- Add the lemon zest, lemon juice and ½ cup of the stock and cook for about 3 minutes or until all the liquid is absorbed, stirring gently.
- Add 1 cup of stock and cook until all the stock is absorbed.
- Stirring occasionally, repeat this process, adding ¾ cup of stock at a time until all the stock is absorbed. (This process will take about 20-30 minutes).
- Stir in the cooked asparagus and the remaining ingredients and cook for about 4 minutes.
- Serve hot.

62) Quinoa and chickpea salad

Preparation time: 15 minutes **Cooking time**: 45 minutes **Portions**: 8

Ingredients:
- 1¾ cups of home-made vegetable stock
- 1 cup quinoa, rinsed
- Sea salt, to taste
- 1½ cups of cooked chickpeas
- 1 medium green pepper, seeded and chopped
- 1 medium red pepper, seeded and chopped

Directions:
- In a pan, add the stock and bring to the boil over high heat.
- Add the quinoa and salt and cook again until boiling.
- Reduce the heat to low and simmer, covered, for about 15-20 minutes or until all the liquid is absorbed.

Ingredients:
- 2 cucumbers, chopped
- ½ cup shallots (only the green part), chopped
- 1 tablespoon olive oil
- 2 tablespoons fresh coriander leaves, chopped

- Remove from the heat and set aside covered for about 5-10 minutes.
- Uncover and stir the quinoa with a fork.
- In a large serving bowl, add the quinoa and remaining ingredients and stir gently to coat.
- Serve immediately.

63) Mixed vegetable soup

Preparation time: **Cooking time**: **Portions**:

Ingredients:
- 1½ tablespoons of olive oil
- 4 medium-sized carrots, peeled and chopped
- 1 medium onion, chopped
- 2 cloves of garlic, minced
- 2 stalks of celery, chopped
- 2 cups fresh tomatoes, finely chopped

Directions:
- In a large soup pot, heat the oil over medium heat and sauté the carrots, celery and onion for 6 minutes.
- Add the garlic and fry for about 1 minute.
- Add the tomatoes and cook for about 2-3 minutes, crushing them with the back of a spoon.

Ingredients:
- 3 cups of small cauliflower florets
- 3 cups of small broccoli florets
- 3 cups frozen peas
- 8 cups of homemade vegetable stock
- 3 tablespoons fresh lemon juice
- Sea salt, to taste

- Add the vegetables and stock and bring to the boil over a high heat.
- Reduce heat to a minimum.
- Cover the pot and simmer for about 30-35 minutes.
- Add the lemon juice and salt and remove from the heat.
- Serve hot.

64) Bean and barley soup

Preparation time: 15 minutes **Cooking time**: 40 minutes **Portions**: 4

Ingredients:
- ✓ 1 tablespoon olive oil
- ✓ 1 white onion, chopped
- ✓ 2 stalks of celery, chopped
- ✓ 1 large carrot, peeled and chopped
- ✓ 2 tablespoons fresh rosemary, chopped
- ✓ 2 cloves of garlic, minced
- ✓ 4 cups fresh tomatoes, chopped

Directions:
- ❖ In a large soup pot, heat the oil over medium heat and sauté the onion, celery and carrot for about 4-5 minutes.
- ❖ Add the garlic and rosemary and fry for about 1 minute.
- ❖ Add the tomatoes and cook for 3-4 minutes, crushing them with the back of a spoon.

Ingredients:
- ✓ 4 cups of homemade vegetable stock
- ✓ 1 cup pearl barley
- ✓ 2 cups of cooked white beans
- ✓ 2 tablespoons fresh lemon juice
- ✓ 4 tablespoons fresh parsley leaves, chopped

- ❖ Add the barley and stock and bring to the boil.
- ❖ Reduce the heat to low and simmer, covered, for about 20-25 minutes.
- ❖ Add the beans and lemon juice and simmer for another 5 minutes or so.
- ❖ Garnish with parsley and serve hot

65) Tofu and pepper stew

Preparation time: 15 minutes   **Cooking time:** 15 minutes   **Portions:** 6

Ingredients:
- ✓ 2 tablespoons of garlic
- ✓ 1 jalapeño pepper, seeded and chopped
- ✓ 1 (16-ounce) can of roasted red peppers, rinsed, drained and chopped
- ✓ 2 cups of homemade vegetable stock
- ✓ 2 cups of filtered water

Directions:
- ❖ Add the garlic, jalapeño pepper and roasted red pepper to a food processor and pulse until smooth.
- ❖ In a large pan, add the puree, stock and water and cook until boiling over medium-high heat.

Ingredients:
- ✓ 1 medium green pepper, seeded and thinly sliced
- ✓ 1 medium red pepper, seeded and thinly sliced
- ✓ 1 (16-ounce) packet of extra-firm tofu, drained and diced
- ✓ 1 (10-ounce) packet of frozen spinach, thawed

- ❖ Add the peppers and tofu and stir to combine.
- ❖ Reduce the heat to medium and cook for about 5 minutes.
- ❖ Stir in the spinach and cook for about 5 minutes.
- ❖ Serve hot.

66) Chickpea stew

Preparation time: 15 minutes   **Cooking time:** 30 minutes   **Portions:** 4

Ingredients:
- ✓ 1 tablespoon olive oil
- ✓ 1 medium onion, chopped
- ✓ 2 cups carrots, peeled and chopped
- ✓ 2 cloves of garlic, minced
- ✓ 1 teaspoon of red pepper flakes
- ✓ 2 large tomatoes, peeled, seeded and finely chopped

Directions:
- ❖ In a large frying pan, heat the oil over medium heat and fry the onion and carrot for about 6 minutes.
- ❖ Add the garlic and red pepper flakes and fry for about 1 minute.
- ❖ Add the tomatoes and cook for about 2-3 minutes.

Ingredients:
- ✓ 2 cups of homemade vegetable stock
- ✓ 2 cups of cooked chickpeas
- ✓ 2 cups fresh spinach, chopped
- ✓ 1 tablespoon fresh lemon juice
- ✓ Sea salt and freshly ground black pepper, to taste

- ❖ Add the stock and bring to the boil.
- ❖ Reduce the heat to low and simmer for about 10 minutes.
- ❖ Stir in the chickpeas and simmer for about 5 minutes.
- ❖ Add the spinach and simmer for a further 3-4 minutes.
- ❖ Add the lemon juice and the seasoning and remove from the heat.
- ❖ Serve hot.

67) Lentils with cabbage

Preparation time: 15 minutes   **Cooking time:** 20 minutes   **Portions: 6**

Ingredients:
- 1½ cups of red lentils
- 1½ cups of home-made vegetable stock
- 1½ tablespoons of olive oil
- ½ cup onion, chopped
- 1 teaspoon fresh ginger, peeled and chopped

Directions:
- In a pan, add the stock and lentils and bring to the boil over medium-high heat.
- Reduce the heat to low and simmer, covered, for about 20 minutes or until almost all the liquid is absorbed.
- Remove from the heat and set aside still covered.

Ingredients:
- 2 cloves of garlic, minced
- 1½ cups tomato, chopped
- 6 cups fresh cabbage, hard ends removed and chopped
- Sea salt and ground black pepper, to taste

- Meanwhile, in a large frying pan, heat the oil over medium heat and fry the onion for about 5-6 minutes.
- Add the ginger and garlic and fry for about 1 minute.
- Add the tomatoes and cabbage and cook for about 4-5 minutes.
- Add the lentils, salt and black pepper and remove from the heat.
- Serve hot.

68) Vegetarian Ratatouille

Preparation time: 20 minutes   **Cooking time:** 45 minutes   **Portions: 4**

Ingredients:
- 6 ounces of homemade tomato paste
- 3 tablespoons of olive oil, divided by
- ½ onion, chopped
- 3 tablespoons minced garlic
- Sea salt and freshly ground black pepper, to taste
- ¾ cup of filtered water
- 1 courgette, cut into thin circles

Directions:
- Preheat the oven to 375 degrees F.
- In a bowl, add the tomato paste, 1 tablespoon of oil, onion, garlic, salt and black pepper and mix well.
- On the bottom of a 10x10 inch baking tray, spread the tomato paste mixture evenly.

Ingredients:
- 1 yellow pumpkin, cut into thin circles
- 1 aubergine, cut into thin circles
- 1 red pepper, seeded and cut into thin circles
- 1 yellow pepper, seeded and cut into thin circles
- 1 tablespoon fresh thyme leaves, chopped
- 1 tablespoon fresh lemon juice

- Arrange the vegetable slices alternately, starting at the outer edge of the pan and working concentrically towards the centre.
- Sprinkle the vegetables with the remaining oil and lemon juice and sprinkle with salt and black pepper and then with thyme.
- Place a piece of parchment paper on top of the vegetables.
- Bake for about 45 minutes.
- Serve hot.

69) Baked beans

Preparation time: 15 minutes   **Cooking time:** 5 hours 5 minutes   **Portions: 4**

Ingredients:
- ¼ pound of dried lima beans, soaked overnight and drained
- ¼ pound of dried red beans, soaked overnight and drained
- 1¼ tablespoons of olive oil
- 1 small yellow onion, chopped
- 4 cloves of garlic, minced
- 1 teaspoon dried thyme, crushed

Directions:
- Add the beans to a large pot of boiling water and bring back to the boil.
- Reduce heat to a minimum.
- Cover the baking tray and bake for about 1 hour.
- Drain the beans well.
- Preheat the oven to 325 degrees F.

Ingredients:
- ½ teaspoon ground cumin
- ½ teaspoon red pepper flakes, crushed
- ¼ teaspoon of smoked paprika
- 1 tablespoon fresh lemon juice
- 1 cup of homemade tomato sauce
- 1 cup of homemade vegetable broth

- In a large oven-proof frying pan, heat the oil over a medium heat and fry the onion for about 4 minutes.
- Add the garlic, thyme and spices and fry for about 1 minute.
- Add the cooked beans and other ingredients and immediately remove from the heat.
- Cover the baking tray and bake in the oven for about 1 hour.
- Serve hot.

70) Barley Pilaf

Preparation time: 20 minutes   **Cooking time:** 1 hour and 5 minutes   **Portions:** 4

Ingredients:
- ½ cup pearl barley
- 1 cup of vegetable stock
- 2 tablespoons of vegetable oil, divided by
- 2 cloves of garlic, minced
- ½ cup white onion, chopped
- ½ cup green olives, sliced

Ingredients:
- ½ cup green pepper, seeded and chopped
- ½ cup of red pepper, seeded and chopped
- 2 tablespoons fresh coriander, chopped
- 2 tablespoons fresh mint leaves, chopped
- 1 tablespoon tamari

Directions:
- In a pan, add the barley and broth over medium-high heat and cook until boiling.
- Immediately, reduce the heat to low and simmer covered for about 45 minutes or until all the liquid has evaporated.
- In a large frying pan, heat 1 tablespoon of oil over medium-high heat and fry the garlic for about 30 seconds.
- Stir in the cooked barley and cook for about 3 minutes.
- Remove from heat and set aside.
- In another pan, heat the remaining oil over medium heat and fry the onion for about 7 minutes.
- Add the olives and peppers and fry for about 3 minutes.
- Stir in the remaining ingredients and cook for about 3 minutes.
- Stir in the barley mixture and cook for about 3 minutes.
- Serve hot.

71) Vegetable and salmon kebabs

Preparation time: **Cooking time:**   **Portions:**

Ingredients:
- 4 wooden skewers
- Pepper (.25 tsp.)
- Salt (.5 tsp.)
- Chopped garlic cloves (1)
- Olive oil (1 tablespoon)
- Sweet onion cut into quarters (.5)
- Sliced yellow pepper (1)
- Cherry Tomatoes (12)
- Chopped courgettes (1)
- Salmon (6 oz.)
- For the plague sauce

Ingredients:
- Pepper (.5 tsp.)
- Salt (1 teaspoon)
- Olive oil (.25 c.)
- Pumpkin seeds (.25 c.)
- Basil leaves (.5 c.)
- Chopped garlic clove (1)
- Spinach (1 c.)
- Lemon juice (1)

Directions:
- Take out the skewers and thread the vegetables and salmon onto them in the way you prefer.
- Place them in a baking dish and then brush them with pepper, garlic, salt and olive oil.
- Turn on the oven and give it time to heat up to 400 degrees. Add the skewers to the oven and bake for a while.
- After 20 minutes, check whether the fish is cooked and then set aside to cool.
- Take out your blender and put in all the ingredients for the pesto sauce. Add more oil if necessary.
- Drizzle the pesto sauce over your salmon skewers before serving.

72) Coconut curry with vegetables

Preparation time: **Cooking time:**   **Portions:**

Ingredients:
- Chopped coriander (3 tbsp)
- Curry powder (2 teaspoons)
- Salt (1 teaspoon)
- Water (.33 c.)
- Coconut milk (1 c.)
- Diced tomato (1)
- Sliced boiled tofu (8 oz)

Ingredients:
- Green beans (.25 lb.)
- Cubed aubergines (.5 c.)
- Sliced yellow pepper (1)
- Diced courgettes (2)
- Diced yellow onion (.5)
- Coconut oil (2 tablespoons)

Directions:
- Take out a frying pan and heat the coconut oil. When the oil is hot, add the beans, aubergines, peppers, courgettes, ginger and onion.
- Cook these for five minutes, and then add the tomatoes and tofu. Stir to cook a little longer.
- After another 5 minutes, add the curry powder, salt, water and coconut milk. Let it simmer for a while.
- Ten minutes later, the dish is ready. Add the coriander and enjoy!

73) Spaghetti squash loaded

Preparation time: **Cooking time:** **Portions:**

Ingredients:
- Lemon peel (.5 tsp.)
- Torn basil leaves (1 c.)
- Salt (.5 tsp.)
- Oregano (.5 tsp.)
- Brown or green lentils, cooked (1 c.)

Directions:
- Turn on the oven and give it time to heat up to 375 degrees. While it heats up, add a little oil to each spaghetti half and then place them face down on a baking sheet lined with baking paper.
- Add the pumpkin to the oven and let it cook until tender. After half an hour, the dish should be ready.
- While this is cooking, heat the rest of the oil in a frying pan. Add the tomatoes, garlic and leeks.

Ingredients:
- Diced tomatoes (6)
- Chopped garlic cloves (1)
- Chopped leek (1)
- Olive oil (1.5 tablespoons)
- Spaghetti squash tagliata (1)

- After eight minutes, you can add the dried oregano and lentils, cooking for another 5 minutes.
- When the pumpkin is ready, remove it from the oven and use a fork to separate the flesh.
- Add the lentil and vegetable mixture to this meat and combine.
- Add the olive oil, lemon zest and torn basil leaves before serving.

74) Spicy pasta

Preparation time: **Cooking time:** **Portions:**

Ingredients:
- Torn basil leaves (1 c.)
- Crushed pepper (1 teaspoon)
- Salt (1 teaspoon)
- Chilli pepper, diced (1)
- Sliced black olives (.5 c.)
- Diced courgettes (.5)
- Dried tomatoes cut into cubes (.5 c.)

Directions:
- Use the instructions on the packet to cook the spelt noodles. Drain the water and set aside.
- Add a little oil to a frying pan before cooking the shallots, carrot, celery and garlic until soft.

Ingredients:
- Diced cherry tomatoes (2 c.)
- Diced carrot (1)
- diced celery stalks (1)
- Shallots, diced (1)
- Chopped garlic cloves (1)
- Olive oil (3 tablespoons)
- Spelt dough (8 oz)

- After eight minutes, add the courgettes, sun-dried tomatoes, cherry tomatoes, pepper, salt, chilli and olives.
- When this is done, throw the pasta into the pan and combine well. Move to a serving dish and cover with a few basil leaves before serving.

75) Stuffed peppers

Preparation time: **Cooking time:** **Portions:**

Ingredients:
- Peppers, cut tops (2)
- Crushed pepper (1 teaspoon)
- Salt (1 teaspoon)
- Chopped coriander (1 tablespoon)
- Lime juice (.5)
- Chilli powder (1 teaspoon)
- Cumin (1 teaspoon)

Directions:
- Take out a bowl and combine the avocado, cucumber, diced pepper, lentils and quinoa.
- In another bowl, whisk together the salt, cilantro, lime juice, chilli, cumin, pepper and olive oil.

Ingredients:
- Olive oil (2 tablespoons)
- Diced avocado (.5)
- Diced cucumber (1)
- Diced red pepper (1)
- Cooked green lentils (.5 c.)
- Cooked quinoa (1 c.)

- Pour this mixture over the lentil and quinoa mixture and mix. Use this mixture to stuff each pepper before serving.

76) *Baba Ganoush Pasta*

Preparation time: **Cooking time:** **Portions:**

Ingredients:
- ✓ Chopped parsley (.25 c.)
- ✓ Cayenne pepper (1 pinch)
- ✓ Salt (.5 tsp.)
- ✓ Vegetable stock (1 tbsp)
- ✓ Chopped chilli pepper (1)
- ✓ Chopped garlic clove (1)
- ✓ Chopped onion (1)

Ingredients:
- ✓ Diced red pepper (.5)
- ✓ Diced courgettes (1)
- ✓ Diced aubergines (1)
- ✓ Olive oil (1 tablespoon)
- ✓ Spelt dough (6 oz)

Directions:
- ❖ Follow the instructions on the packet to cook the spelt pasta and then set it aside.
- ❖ Heat some oil in a frying pan and when the oil is ready, add the chilli, garlic, onion, pepper, courgettes and aubergines to the pan.
- ❖ After 6 minutes of cooking, add the vegetable stock and cook for a further 5 minutes or until hot.
- ❖ Remove it from the oven and leave it to cool for a few minutes before adding it to the blender. Blend until nice and smooth.
- ❖ Add the sauce to your pan and season with a little pepper and salt. Add the cooked pasta and sprinkle with parsley before serving.

77) *Broccoli bowl with cheese*

Preparation time: **Cooking time:** **Portions:**

Ingredients:
- ✓ Crushed black pepper (.5 tsp.)
- ✓ Salt (.5 tsp.)
- ✓ Yeast feeding (.24 c.)
- ✓ Lemon juice (1 tablespoon)

Ingredients:
- ✓ Cooked broccoli florets (4 c.)
- ✓ Cooked quinoa (1 c.)
- ✓ Olive oil (1 tablespoon)

Directions:
- ❖ To start this recipe, take out a frying pan and add the oil, broccoli and cooked quinoa.
- ❖ Remove the dish from the heat and serve hot.
- ❖ After five minutes, this should be nice and hot, then add the pepper, salt, nutritional yeast and lemon juice.

78) *Green bean and lentil salad*

Preparation time: **Cooking time:** **Portions:**

Ingredients:
- ✓ Shallot (2 tablespoons)
- ✓ Apple cider vinegar (.25 c.)
- ✓ Sliced green beans (2 c.)
- ✓ Halved cherry tomatoes (1 c.)
- ✓ Cooked green lentils (2 c.)
- ✓ Pesto sauce

Ingredients:
- ✓ Salt (1 teaspoon)
- ✓ Olive oil (.25 c.)
- ✓ Chopped garlic clove (1)
- ✓ Pine nuts (2 tablespoons)
- ✓ Spinach (.5 c.)
- ✓ Basil leaves (.75 c.)

Directions:
- ❖ Take out the food processor and add all the ingredients for the pesto sauce to make it creamy and smooth.
- ❖ In another bowl, combine the vinegar, green beans, tomatoes, lentils and shallots.
- ❖ Pour the pesto sauce over the mixture in the bowl, stir to coat and then serve.

79) Vegetable soup

Preparation time:
Cooking time:
Portions:

Ingredients:
- Spinach (1 c.)
- Basil (1c)
- Pepper (1 teaspoon)
- Salt (2 teaspoons)
- Oregano (1 tablespoon)
- Diced tomatoes (1 c.)
- Vegetable stock (1 tbsp)
- Kidney beans (.5 c.)

Ingredients:
- Chopped garlic clove (1)
- Shallot (1)
- Diced carrot (.5 c.)
- Diced courgettes (.5 c.)
- Diced pumpkin (.5 c.)
- Cubed aubergines (.5 c.)
- Olive oil (1 tablespoon)

Directions:
- Take out a stock pot and heat the olive oil in it. When the oil is hot, add the garlic, shallot, carrot, courgette, pumpkin and aubergine to the pot.
- After five minutes of cooking, add salt, oregano, diced tomatoes, stock, beans and pepper.
- Let these ingredients simmer for another ten minutes, adding more spices if desired.
- Add the spinach and basil just before serving and enjoy.

80) South West Hamburger

Preparation time:
Cooking time:
Portions:

Ingredients:
- Sliced avocado (1)
- Lettuce leaves, Bibb (2)
- Rocket (1c)
- Dijon mustard (1 tablespoon)
- Crushed walnuts (1 tablespoon)
- Nutritional yeast (1 tablespoon)
- Boiled tofu (4 oz)
- Crushed black pepper (.5 tsp.)
- Cayenne pepper (.5 tsp.)

Ingredients:
- Ground cumin (1 teaspoon)
- Salt (1 teaspoon)
- Diced carrot (1)
- Diced green pepper (1 c.)
- Diced yellow onion (5.)
- Olive oil (1 tablespoon)

Directions:
- Heat oil in a frying pan. When the oil is hot, add the onion, pepper, cayenne, cumin, salt, carrot and pepper.
- After five minutes, the vegetables should be soft. Pour them into a bowl and leave to cool.
- Grate the tofu over the bowl and then add the Dijon mustard, walnuts and nutritional yeast. Mix everything together well and form two burgers.
- Turn on the oven and let it heat up to 400 degrees. Place the burgers on a paper-lined baking tray and then put them in the oven.
- After half an hour, the burgers should be ready. Remove from the oven and leave to cool before topping with avocado and serving.

81) Courgette rolls with red sauce

Preparation time: **Cooking time:** **Portions:**

Ingredients:
- Basil leaves (15)
- Sliced courgettes (2)
- Water (.75 c.)
- Dried oregano (1 teaspoon)
- Salt (1 teaspoon)
- Diced red pepper (1)
- Diced Roma tomatoes (3)
- Chopped yellow onion (1)
- Olive oil (1 tablespoon)

Directions:
- Take out a frying pan and heat some oil in it. Add the oregano, salt, pepper, tomato and onion to make your red vegetable mixture.
- Cook for a few minutes to make the vegetables soft, and then add a little water. Let it simmer for a while.
- After ten minutes, remove the pan from the heat and give the vegetable mixture time to cool.
- Transfer to a blender and blend until smooth.

Ingredients:
- Basil filling
- Chopped basil (1 handful)
- Nutmeg (.25 tsp.)
- Crushed pepper (.25 tsp.)
- Salt (.5 tsp.)
- Nutritional yeast (1 tablespoon)
- Water (3 tablespoons)
- Lemon juice (1)
- Soaked cashews (1 c.)

- Now, work on the cashew nut filling. Clean the food processor and add all the ingredients until you get a smooth dough. This can take some time, so be patient while doing it.
- Place the courgette ribbons on a plate in front of you and divide the filling between each one. Roll up each ribbon tightly and then place it in an oven dish with the red vegetable mixture at the bottom.
- Cover each of these rolls with the rest of the red vegetable mixture and add to the oven which is heated to 375 degrees.
- After 15 minutes, remove the tray from the oven and leave the dish to cool. Before serving, place the basil leaves on top and enjoy.

82) Meatless Taco Wraps

Preparation time: **Cooking time:** **Portions:**

Ingredients:
- Avocado slices (.5)
- Romaine leaves (4)
- Water (.25 c.)
- Salt (.5 tsp.)
- Cumin (.5 tsp.)
- Chilli powder (.5 tsp.)
- Smoked paprika (.5 tsp.)
- Chopped garlic clove (1)
- Tomato paste (1 tablespoon)
- Roasted walnuts (.5 c.)

Directions:
- Start with the sauce. Add all the ingredients in a bowl and stir to combine. Let marinate for a while while you work on your taco "meat".

Ingredients:
- Cooked brown lentils (1.5 c.)
- For the sauce
- Crushed pepper (.5 tsp.)
- Salt (.5 tsp.)
- Apple cider vinegar (1 tablespoon)
- Chopped coriander (3 tbsp)
- Diced green pepper (.5 c.)
- Diced red pepper (.5 c.)
- Diced mango (.5 c.)

- Take out the food processor and put together the water, salt, cumin, chilli powder, paprika, garlic, tomato paste, walnuts and lentils. You want this to still be a bit crumbly when you're done.
- Place the walnut and lentil mixture in each romaine lettuce leaf, and then cover with the sauce and avocado slices before serving.

83) Sesame and quinoa pilaf

Preparation time: **Cooking time:**   **Portions:**

Ingredients:
- Cooked green lentils (1 c.)
- Broth or water (1 c.)
- Quinoa (.5 c.)
- Chopped garlic clove (1)
- Diced green pepper (.5 c.)
- Celery stalk, diced (1)
- Sliced shallot (1)
- Crushed pepper (2 teaspoons)
- Salt (2 teaspoons)
- Olive oil (2 tablespoons)
- Sliced carrots (2)

Ingredients:
- Green beans cut and sliced (1 c.)
- For the dressing
- Black sesame seeds (2 tablespoons)
- Rice vinegar (.25 c.)
- Tamari (.25 c.)
- Red pepper flakes (.5 tsp.)
- Lemon peel (1 teaspoon)
- Grated ginger (1 teaspoon)
- Toasted sesame oil (2 tablespoons)
- Avocado oil (.33 c.)

Directions:
- Place the carrots and green beans on baking paper on a baking tray. Sprinkle with pepper, salt and a tablespoon of olive oil.
- Add to the grill of the oven and bake until golden brown. This will take about five minutes.
- Once this is done, take a pot and add the garlic, pepper, celery, shallot and the rest of the oil.
- Cook the ingredients for five minutes before adding the quinoa and stirring to cook a little longer.
- Now add the water or broth and bring to the boil. Let it simmer for a while until the liquid has disappeared.
- Now you can prepare the dressing. To do this, whisk all the ingredients in a bowl to combine them.
- When it's time to assemble, mix together the quinoa and lentils. Season with a little pepper and salt and then add the carrot and bean mixture before pouring the dressing over everything.

SNACKs

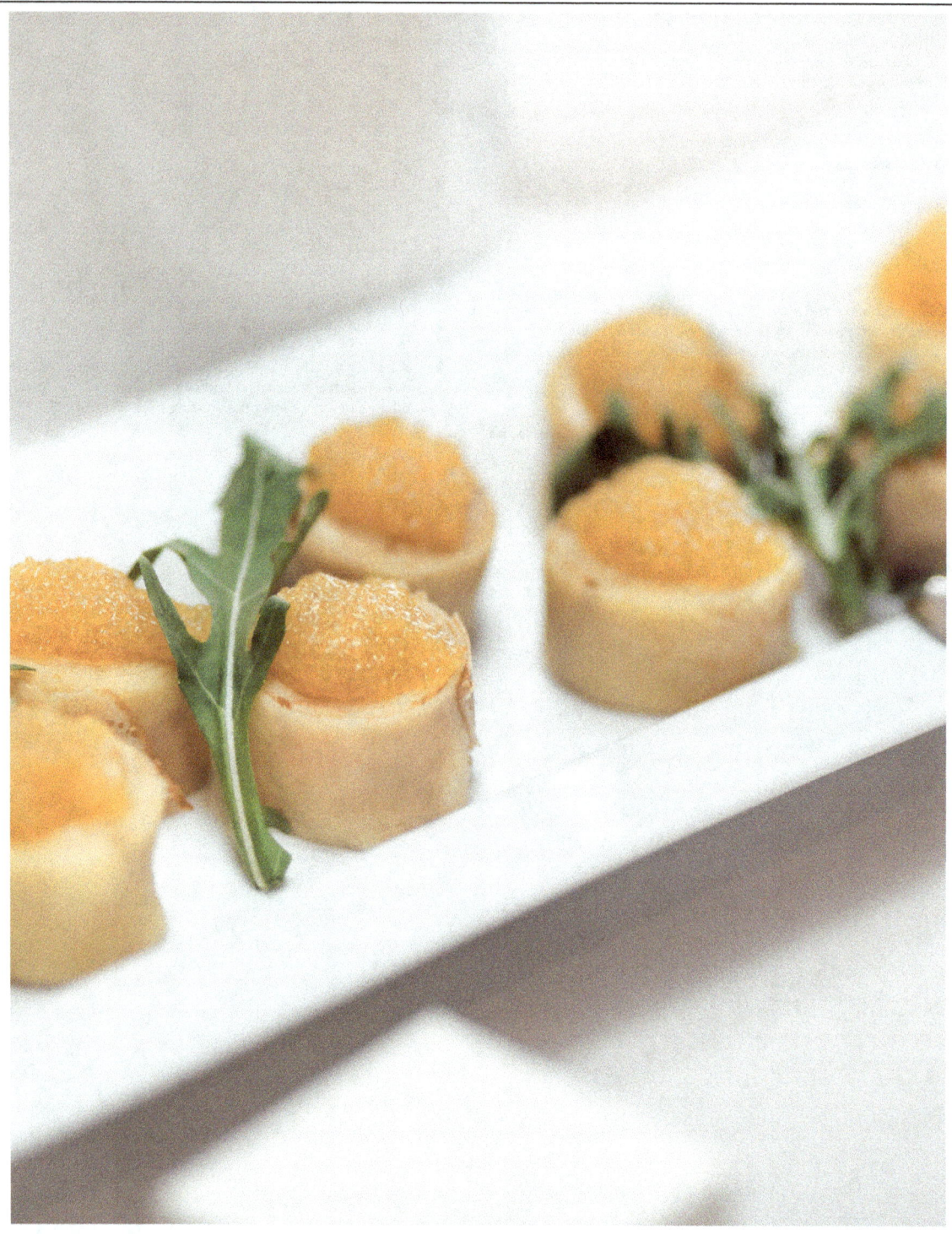

84) Aloo Gobi

Preparation time:

Cooking time:

Servings: 1 bowl

Ingredients:
- ✓ Cauliflower, 750g
- ✓ Fresh ginger, 20g
- ✓ Large onions, 2
- ✓ Mint, 1/3 cup
- ✓ Turmeric, 2 teaspoons
- ✓ Diced tomatoes, 400g
- ✓ Fresh garlic, 2 cloves
- ✓ Cayenne pepper, 2 teaspoons

Ingredients:
- ✓ Cilantro/coriander leaves, 1/3 cup
- ✓ Large potatoes, 4
- ✓ Garam masala, 2 teaspoons
- ✓ Green chilli, 4
- ✓ Water, 3 cups
- ✓ Extra virgin olive oil (cold pressed), 125 ml
- ✓ Salt to taste

Directions:
- ❖ Blend the chilli, garlic and ginger.
- ❖ Fry the oil in a wok for three minutes and add the onion until golden brown.
- ❖ Add the ground pasta and fry for a few seconds, then add; garam masala, chilli, turmeric, tomatoes and salt.
- ❖ Cook for about five minutes and add all the other ingredients.
- ❖ Stir for three minutes and add the water.
- ❖ Cook until the sauce is thick.
- ❖ Serve with Basmati rice or as a side dish.

85) Chocolate Crunch Bars

Preparation time: 3 hours

Cooking time: 5 minutes

Portions: 4

Ingredients:
- ✓ 1 1/2 cups sugar-free chocolate chips
- ✓ 1 cup of nut butter
- ✓ Stevia for taste

Ingredients:
- ✓ 1/4 cup of coconut oil
- ✓ 3 cups pecans, chopped

Directions:
- ❖ Prepare an 8-inch baking tray with baking paper.
- ❖ Mix chips chocolate with butter, coconut oil and sweetener in a bowl.
- ❖ Melt in the microwave for 2 to 3 minutes until melted.
- ❖ Add the cube and nuts. Stir gently.
- ❖ Put this stick in the oven and it will never open again.
- ❖ Refrigerate for 2 to 3 hours.
- ❖ Slice and serve.

86) Walnut butter Bars

Preparation time: 40 minutes.

Cooking time: 10 minutes.

Portions: 6

Ingredients:
- ✓ 3/4 cup of walnut flour
- ✓ 2 ounces of nut butter
- ✓ 1/4 cup Swerve

Ingredients:
- ✓ 1/2 wooden walnut
- ✓ 1/2 teaspoon vanilla

Directions:
- ❖ Combine all the ingredients for a better result.
- ❖ Transfer the contents to a small 6-inch baking tin. Press firmly.
- ❖ Refrigerate for 30 minutes.
- ❖ Cut into slices and serve.

87) Homemade Protein Bar

Preparation time: 5 mnutes

Cooking time: 10 minutes

Portions: 4

Ingredients:
- ✓ 1 knob of butter
- ✓ 4 tbsp. coconut oil
- ✓ 2 scoops of vanilla protein

Ingredients:
- ✓ To taste, ½ tsp of sea salt Optional Ingredients:
- ✓ 1 teaspoon cinnamon

Directions:
- ❖ Mix coconut oil with butter, protein, stevia and salt in a dish.
- ❖ Mix cinnamon and chocolate chips.
- ❖ Presss the dough is firmly and freezed until firmed.
- ❖ Cut the crust into small bars.
- ❖ Serve and enjoy.

88) Shortbread Coookies

Preparation time: 10 minutes **Cooking time**: 1 hour and 10 minutes **Portions**: 6

Ingredients:
- 2 1/2 cups coconut flour
- 6 tablespoons of nut butter

Directions:
- Preheat our oven to 350 degrees.
- Place on a biscuit sheet with the parchment paper.
- Beat the butter with the erythritol until frothy.
- Add the vanilla essence and coconut flour.

Ingredients:
- 1/2 cup erythritol
- 1 teaspoon of vanilla essence

- Stir until crumbling.
- Spoon out a tablespoon of cookie dough onto the cookie sheet.
- Add more dough to make a pile.
- Bake for 15 minutes until golden brown.
- Serve.

89) Coconut biscuits Chip

Preparation time: 10 minutes **Cooking time**: 15 minutes **Portions**: 4

Ingredients:
- 1 cup of walnut flour
- ½ cup cacao nibs
- ½ cup coconut flakes, unsweetened
- 1/3 cup erythritol
- ½ cup nut butter

Directions:
- Prepare the oven for 350 degrees F.
- Layer a cookie sheet with parchment paper.
- Add and combine all the ingredients dry in a glass bowl.
- Coconut milk, vanilla, stevia and peanut butter.
- Beating well stir in the battery. Mix well.

Ingredients:
- ¼ cup peanut launcher, more than once
- ¼ cup of coconut milk
- Stevia, as desired
- ¼ teaspoon of sea salt

- Spoon out a tablespoon of cookie dough on the coookie sheet.
- Add more dough to make 16 coookies.
- Fluctuate each cookie using your fingers.
- Water for 25 minutes until dawn.
- Let them rest for 15 minutes.
- Serve.

90) Coconut Cookies

Preparation time: 10 mnutes **Cooking time**: 20 minutes **Portions**: 6

Ingredients:
- 6 tablespoons coconut flour
- ¾ teaspoons baking powder
- 1/8 teaspoon sea salt
- 3 tablespoons of nut butter

Directions:
- Preheat our oven to 375 degrees F. Layer a biscuit sheet with parchment.
- Place all the wet ingredients in a blender. Blend all the mixture in a blender.
- Add the wet mixture and mix well until it is absorbed.

Ingredients:
- 1/6 cup coconut oil
- 6 tablespoon data sugar
- 1/3 cup coco nut milk
- 1/2 teaspoon vanilla essence

- Place a spoonful of dough cookie on the biscuit sheet.
- Add a little more butter to make many coookies. Bake until golden brown (about 10 minutes). We will see.

91) Berry Mousse

Preparation time: 5 minutes **Cooking time**: 5 minutes **Portions**: 2

Ingredients:
- 1 teaspoon Seville orange zest
- 3 oz. raspberries or blueberries.

Directions:
- Blend the rice in an electric blender until the fluff is dissolved.
- Add the vanilla and Seville zest. Stir well.
- Add the nuts and berries.

Ingredients:
- ¼ teaspoon vanilla essence
- 2 cups coconut cream

- Cover the glove with a plastic key.
- Refrigerate for 3 hours.
- Garnish as desired. Serve.

92) Coconut pulp Coookies

Preparation time: 5 minutes. **Cooking time:** 10 hours. **Portions:** 4

Ingredients:
- ✓ 3 cups coconut pulp
- ✓ 1 Granny Smith apple
- ✓ 1-2 teaspoon cinnamon

Directions:
- ❖ Blend the coconut with the remaining ingredients in a processor food.
- ❖ Make many biscuits with this mixture.
- ❖ Place them on a kitchen table, lined with parchment.

Ingredients:
- ✓ 2-3 tablespoons of raw honey
- ✓ 1/4 cup coco walnut flakes

- ❖ Place the dough in a food oven for 6-10 hours at 115 degrees Fahrenheit.
- ❖ Serve.

93) Avocado Pudding

Preparation time: 10 minutes **Cooking time:** 0 minutes **Portions:** 2

Ingredients:
- ✓ 2 avocados
- ✓ 3/4-1 cup coconut milk
- ✓ 1/3-1/2 cup of raw cacao powder

Directions:
- ❖ Mix all ingredients in a blender.

Ingredients:
- ✓ 1 teaspoon 100% pure organic vanilla (optional)
- ✓ 2-4 tablespoons of date sugar

- ❖ Refrigerate for 4 hours in a container.
- ❖ Serve.

94) Coconut Raisins cooookies

Preparation time: 10 minutes. **Cooking time:** 10 minutes. **Portions:** 4

Ingredients:
- ✓ 1 1/4 cups coconut flour 1 cup nut flour
- ✓ 1 teaspoon baking soda
- ✓ 1/2 Celtic teaspoon sea salt
- ✓ 1 peanut button cup
- ✓ 1 cup coconut date sugar

Directions:
- ❖ Turn on the oven to 357 degrees F.
- ❖ Mix the flour with the salt and baking soda.
- ❖ Flatten with sugar until you start and then stirs in walnut milk and vinavilla.

Ingredients:
- ✓ 2 teaspoons of vanilla
- ✓ ¼ cup coconut milk
- ✓ 3/4 cup organic sultanas
- ✓ 3/4 cup coconut chips or flakes

- ❖ Mix well, then place in a container for the powder. Stir until fine.
- ❖ Add all remaining ingredients.
- ❖ Make small coookies out this dough.
- ❖ Place the biscuits on a baking tray.
- ❖ Bake for 10 minutes until set.

95) Cracker Pumpkin Spice

Preparation time: 10 minutes. **Cooking time:** 1 hour. **Portions:** 6

Ingredients:
- ✓ 1/3 cup coco walnut flour
- ✓ 2 tablespoons pumpkin pie spice
- ✓ ¾ cup sunflower seds
- ✓ ¾ cup flaxseed
- ✓ 1/3 cup sesame seeds

Directions:
- ❖ Heat our oven to 300 degrees F. Combine all ingredients in a bowl.
- ❖ Add the salt and oil to the mixture and mix well.
- ❖ Let the dough rest for 2 to 3 minutes.

Ingredients:
- ✓ 1 tablespoon gron psyllium husk powder
- ✓ 1 teaspoon sea salt
- ✓ 3 tablespoons coco walnut oil, melted
- ✓ 1 1/3 cups water

- ❖ Roll out the dough on a cookie sheet lined with parchment paper.
- ❖ Bake for 30 minutes.
- ❖ Reduce the amount of food to 30 m and let it rest for another 30 m.
- ❖ Crush the bread into small pieces. Serve

96) Spicy Toasted nuts

Preparation time: 10 minutes. **Cooking time:** 15 minutes. **Portions: 4**

Ingredients:
- 8 ounces of pecans or coconuts or walnuts
- 1 teaspoon sea salt
- 1 tablespoon olive oil or coconut oil

Directions:
- Add all the ingredients to an oven. Fry the nuts until golden brown.

Ingredients:
- 1 teaspoon of ground cumin
- 1 teaspoon paprika powder or chili powder

- Serve and enjoy.

DESSERTS

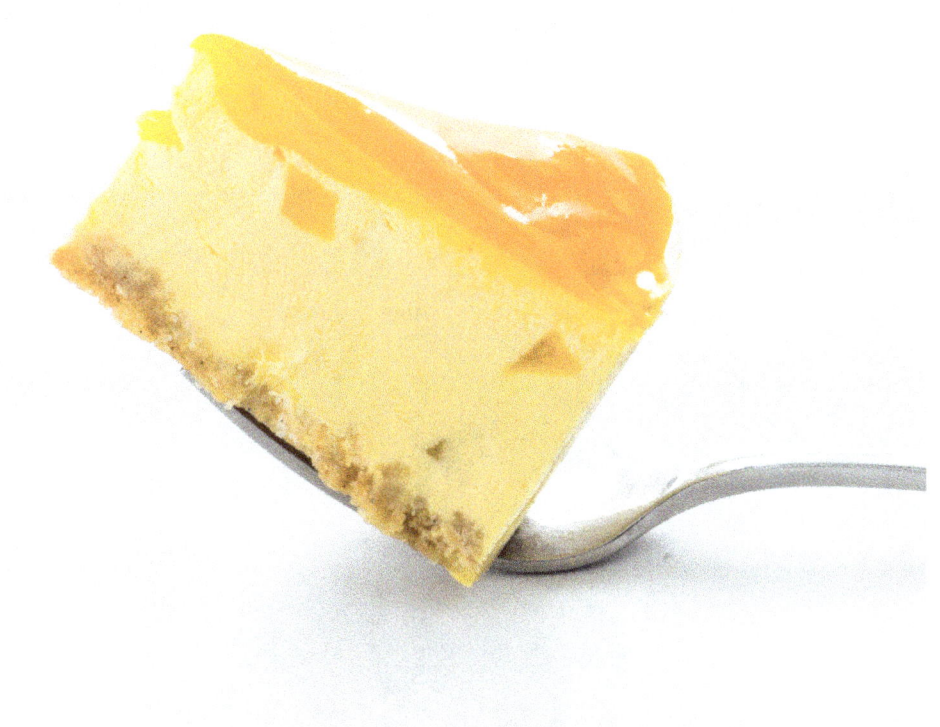

97) Cabbage and pineapple smoothie

Preparation time: 15 minutes **Cooking time**: **Portions**: 2

Ingredients:
- 1½ cups fresh cabbage, chopped and shredded
- 1 frozen banana, peeled and chopped
- ½ cup of fresh pineapple chunks

Directions:
- Add all ingredients to a high-speed blender and pulse until smooth.

Ingredients:
- 1 cup unsweetened coconut milk
- ½ cup of fresh orange juice
- ½ cup of ice
- Pour the smoothie into two glasses and serve immediately.

98) Green vegetable smoothie

Preparation time: 15 minutes **Cooking time**: **Portions**: 2

Ingredients:
- 1 medium avocado, peeled, pitted and chopped
- 1 large cucumber, peeled and chopped
- 2 fresh tomatoes, chopped
- 1 small green pepper, seeded and chopped

Directions:
- Add all ingredients to a high-speed blender and pulse until smooth.

Ingredients:
- 1 cup fresh spinach, torn
- 2 tablespoons fresh lime juice
- 2 tablespoons of homemade vegetable stock
- 1 cup of alkaline water
- Pour the smoothie into glasses and serve immediately.

99) Avocado and spinach smoothie

Preparation time: 10 minutes **Cooking time**: **Portions**: 2

Ingredients:
- 2 cups of fresh spinach
- ½ avocado, peeled, pitted and chopped
- 4-6 drops of liquid stevia

Directions:
- Add all ingredients to a high-speed blender and pulse until smooth.

Ingredients:
- ½ teaspoon ground cinnamon
- 1 tablespoon hemp seeds
- 2 cups of cooled alkaline water
- Pour the smoothie into two glasses and serve immediately.

100) Cucumber smoothie

Preparation time: 15 minutes **Cooking time**: **Portions**: 2

Ingredients:
- 1 small cucumber, peeled and chopped
- 2 cups of fresh mixed vegetables (spinach, cabbage, chard), chopped and shredded
- ½ cup of lettuce, torn
- ¼ cup of fresh parsley leaves
- ¼ cup of fresh mint leaves

Directions:
- Add all ingredients to a high-speed blender and pulse until smooth.

Ingredients:
- 2-3 drops of liquid stevia
- 1 teaspoon fresh lemon juice
- 1½ cups of filtered water
- ¼ cup ice cubes

- Pour the smoothie into two glasses and serve immediately.

101) Apple and ginger smoothie

Preparation time: 10 minutes **Cooking time**: 0 minutes **Portions**: 1

Ingredients:
- 1 apple, peeled and diced
- ¾ cup (6 oz) of coconut yoghurt

Directions:
- Add all ingredients to a blender.
- Blend well until smooth.

Ingredients:
- ½ teaspoon of freshly grated ginger

- Refrigerate for 2 to 3 hours.
- Serve.

102) Blueberry smoothie with green tea

Preparation time: 10 minutes **Cooking time**: 5 minutes **Portions**: 1

Ingredients:
- 3 tablespoons of alkaline water
- 1 green tea bag
- 1½ cups of fresh blueberries

Directions:
- Boil 3 tablespoons of water in a small saucepan and transfer to a cup.
- Immerse the tea bag in the cup and let it stand for 4 to 5 minutes.
- Discard the tea bag and
- Transfer green tea into a blender

Ingredients:
- 1 pear, peeled, stoned and diced
- ¾ cup of almond milk

- Add all other ingredients to the blender.
- Blend well until smooth.
- Serve with fresh blueberries.

103) Apple and almond smoothie

Preparation time: 10 minutes **Cooking time**: 0 minutes **Portions: 1**

Ingredients:
- 1 cup of apple cider
- 1/2 cup of coconut yoghurt
- 4 tablespoons almonds, crushed

Ingredients:
- 1/4 teaspoon of cinnamon
- 1/4 teaspoon nutmeg
- 1 cup of ice cubes

Directions:
- Add all ingredients to a blender.
- Blend well until smooth.
- Serve.

104) Cranberry smoothie

Preparation time: 10 minutes **Cooking time**: 0 minutes **Portions: 1**

Ingredients:
- 1 cup cranberries
- ¾ cup of almond milk
- ¼ cup raspberries

Ingredients:
- 2 teaspoons fresh ginger, finely grated
- 2 teaspoons of fresh lemon juice

Directions:
- Add all ingredients to a blender.
- Blend well until smooth.
- Serve with fresh berries on top.

105) Berry and cinnamon smoothie

Preparation time: 10 minutes **Cooking time**: 0 minutes **Portions: 1**

Ingredients:
- 1 cup frozen strawberries
- 1 cup apple, peeled and diced
- 2 teaspoons of fresh ginger
- 3 tablespoons of hemp seeds

Ingredients:
- 1 cup of water
- ½ lime, squeezed
- ¼ teaspoon cinnamon powder
- ⅛ teaspoon of vanilla extract

Directions:
- Add all ingredients to a blender.
- Blend well until smooth.
- Serve with fresh fruit

106) Detoxifying berry smoothie

Preparation time: 10 minutes **Cooking time**: 0 minutes **Portions: 1**

Ingredients:
- 3 peaches, with stone and skin
- 5 blueberries

Ingredients:
- 5 raspberries
- 1 cup of alkaline water

Directions:
- Add all ingredients to a blender.
- Blend well until smooth.
- Serve with fresh kiwi slices.

107) Pink smoothie

Preparation time: 10 minutes **Cooking time:** 0 minutes **Portions: 1**

Ingredients:
- 1 peach, core and skin
- 6 ripe strawberries

Ingredients:
- 1 cup of almond milk

Directions:
- Add all ingredients to a blender.
- Blend well until smooth.
- Serve with your favourite berries

108) Green apple smoothie

Preparation time: 10 minutes **Cooking time:** 0 minutes **Portions: 1**

Ingredients:
- 1 peach, peeled and pitted
- 1 green apple, peeled and cored

Ingredients:
- 1 cup of alkaline water

Directions:
- Add all ingredients to a blender.
- Blend well until smooth.
- Serve with apple slices.

PART 2- INTRODUCTION TO THE ALKALINE DIET

Each specific diet plan for health is created to produce somewhat similar results, but each follows a different path to achieve those goals. Experts developed the Alkaline Diet to help our bodies work effectively and efficiently, curbing the threats of many diseases. This is because the human body requires an optimal pH level for all enzymes to function effectively. The neutrality of the internal environment can only be maintained with a good and balanced diet. Since most foods are more acidic, we all suffer from intestinal acidity, indigestion, and other related diseases. The alkaline diet can solve all these problems as it offers a proper approach to maintain the internal pH level.

Let's start with a bit of review of our chemistry lessons and remember what pH is. A simple definition is how much concentration of hydrogen ions there is in our body. The acronym pH is an abbreviation for "hydrogen potency." The "p" stands for "potent" or the German word for power, and "H" stands for the symbol for the element hydrogen. The pH scale ranges from 1 to 14. Seven is neutral. A pH below seven is acidic. Solutions that have a pH above seven are alkaline.

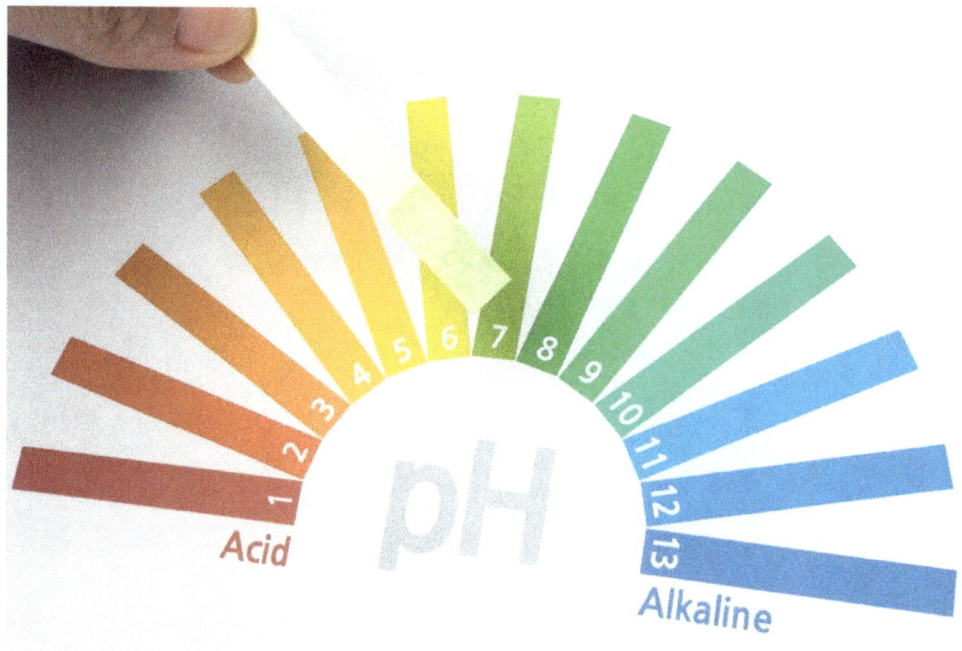

To have good health, our bodies must be somewhat alkaline. The pH of our blood and other cellular fluids should be around a pH between 7.365 and 7.45. It is essential to understand that pH levels vary significantly throughout the body. Some parts will be acidic, while others will be alkaline. There is no set level. For example, our stomach is loaded with hydrochloric acid, giving it a pH of between 2 and 3.5. This makes it very acidic. It needs to be so acidic to break down the foods we consume and kill harmful bacteria. Our saliva has a pH between 6.8 and 7.3. The skin has a pH level of 4 to 6.5. This acts as a protective barrier from the environment. Our urine has a pH that ranges from alkaline to acidic. It all depends on what you eat.

The most critical measure is the pH of your blood. It needs to stay in a very narrow range between 7.365 and 7.45. This may sound simple, but instead of operating on a mathematical scale, our pH operates on a logarithmic scale in multiples of ten. This means that it will take ten times the amount of alkalinity to neutralize an acid. A pH of five will be 100 times more acidic than a pH of seven. A pH of four will be 1,000 times more acidic. Does this help you understand?

Don't start stressing about being in or out of this range. Remember that our bodies are pretty good at regulating the pH of our blood. However, our bodies don't "find" the balance. It has many parts that do, and it keeps the pH of your blood between 7.365 and 7.45 at all times. If you make poor lifestyle and food choices, your body works harder to maintain balance. If you want to address inflammation and acidity in your body by changing your food choices to more alkaline foods, this will help balance your system and return your body to its best vitality.

BLOOD pH

You know that the body is constantly working to maintain healthy pH levels in your body. The tricky thing is that three fluids in the body are typically at slightly different pH levels. But, overall, they are mainly controlled by the same things. So the first thing we're going to look at is the pH of the blood.

The normal pH range for blood is 7.35 to 7.45. This means that the blood usually is alkaline or basic by nature. However, compared to stomach acid, which is between 3 and 5.5, you can see a big difference. The stomach is supposed to be at this acidic level to break down the food you eat. Ironically, if your stomach acid becomes more acidic or more basic, it can create the same symptoms of acid reflux, but that's another matter. This low pH helps you digest your food and destroys germs that may enter your stomach.

What can cause your blood pH to change or reach abnormal levels?

Health problems are usually the most common cause of your blood becoming too alkaline or acidic. In addition, a change in normal blood pH levels can signal a medical emergency or health condition. This may include:

- Poisoning
- Drug overdose
- Bleeding
- Shock
- Infection
- Gout
- Lung disease
- Kidney disease
- Heart disease
- Diabetes
- Asthma

Acidosis refers to when the blood pH level drops below 7.35 and begins to become too acidic. Alkalosis refers to when the pH level of the blood increases to more than 7.45 and starts to become too alkaline. Two main organs work hard to help maintain normal pH levels in the blood:

- Kidneys - These organs work to remove acid through urine to excrete it.
- Lungs - These organs work by getting rid of carbon dioxide through breathing.

The different forms of blood alkalosis and acidosis depend significantly on the cause. However, the two leading causes are:

- Metabolic - These types of problems occur most often when the pH of the blood changes due to a problem with a condition in the kidneys.
- Respiratory - These types of problems occur most often when the blood pH changes due to a respiratory or pulmonary condition.

It is common for blood pH levels to be tested as part of a blood gas test. This type of test is also called an ABG test or arterial blood gas test. It works by measuring how much carbon dioxide and oxygen are in your blood. Your general practitioner may choose to test your blood pH as a regular part of your annual health screenings or if you already have certain health conditions. Blood pH tests require blood to be drawn with a needle. The lab will receive the blood sample and perform the test.

There are at-home blood pH tests that you can do by pricking your finger. These tests will not give you an accurate reading like a test in your doctor's office. Using a urine pH test will not show you the pH level of your blood, but it can let you know if something is wrong.

Let's take a moment to take a closer look at some reasons why your blood pH levels move outside of the normal range.

High blood pH, also known as alkalosis, occurs if the pH of your blood rises above the normal range. There are many reasons for high blood pH levels. For example, you can have a temporary increase in blood pH with simple illnesses. Certain foods can also cause your blood to become more alkaline. However, there are also more serious causes for this alkalosis that can create additional problems.

The first is fluid loss. Losing too much water can cause the pH levels in your blood to rise. This is because you also lose some electrolytes in your blood, minerals, and salts when you lose water. These include potassium and sodium. In addition, diarrhea, vomiting, and sweating can cause excess fluid loss.

Medications and diuretics can also cause a person to urinate more often, leading to increased pH levels in the blood. Treatment for fluid loss requires making sure you are getting plenty of fluids and replacing electrolytes. Some sports drinks can be used for this purpose. Your doctor can also review your medications and stop those that may be causing fluid loss.

Next, kidney problems can cause high pH levels in the blood. The kidneys play an essential role in maintaining normal blood pH. Therefore, a kidney problem can cause a buildup of alkalinity in the blood. This is because the kidneys do not remove excess alkaline substances through the urine. For example, the kidneys may improperly filter bicarbonate in the blood. Medications can regulate it.

When there is acidosis in the blood, it can affect how every organ in your body works. Low blood pH is a more common problem than high blood pH. Acidosis is often a warning sign of some health problem that is not being controlled.

Some health conditions can cause natural acids to build up in the blood. Some forms of acids that can end up lowering the pH of the blood include:

- Carbonic acid

- Hydrochloric acid

- Phosphoric acid

- Sulfuric acid

- Ketogenic acids

- Lactic acid

An improper diet can cause problems. Eating an unbalanced diet can create a temporary low pH level in the blood. Not eating enough or going for long periods without eating can make more acid in the blood. Try to avoid eating too many acid-forming foods, which include:

- Grains - rice, pasta, bread, and flour

- fish

- Meat

- Eggs

- Poultry - turkey and chicken

- Dairy products - yogurt, cheese, and cow's milk

Balance your blood pH by eating more alkaline foods. These more often include dried, frozen, and fresh fruits and fresh and cooked vegetables. Stay away from fad or starvation diets. Instead, when trying to lose weight, do so healthily and safely by following a balanced diet.

Another cause of low blood pH levels is due to diabetic ketoacidosis. If you have diabetes, your blood can end up becoming acidic if you don't regulate your blood sugar levels properly. Diabetic ketoacidosis occurs when your body can't make enough insulin or use it properly.

Insulin helps move sugar from the foods we eat into the cells of the body. This is where the body burns it as fuel. If insulin cannot be used, the body begins to break down the fat stored in the body for fuel. This releases a wasted acid known as ketones. If the body cannot regulate this process, the acid will build up and trigger a low pH in the blood.

You must seek emergency care if your blood sugar level exceeds 300 milligrams per deciliter. If you suffer from any of the following symptoms, talk to your doctor:

- Confusion
- Stomach pain
- Shortness of breath
- Shortness of breath
- Vomiting or nausea
- Weakness or fatigue
- Frequent urination
- Excessive thirst

Diabetic ketoacidosis is most often a sign that diabetes is not being treated properly and is out of control. This can sometimes be the first sign of diabetes for some people. Making sure your diabetes is well treated will help keep your blood pH in balance. It may require a strict diet and exercise plan, insulin injections, and medications to stay healthy.

The third cause of low blood pH is metabolic acidosis. This is when low blood pH is caused by kidney disease or failure. This occurs when the kidneys fail in removing acids from the body through urination. This will increase the acids in your body and lower your blood pH.

The most common symptoms of metabolic acidosis include.

- Heavy breathing
- Fast heartbeat
- Headaches
- Vomiting and nausea
- Loss of appetite
- Weakness and fatigue

Treatment for this problem often includes medications to help the kidneys work better, but a kidney transplant or dialysis is the only solution for severe cases. Dialysis works by cleansing the blood.

The final cause of low pH in the blood is respiratory acidosis. When the lungs are probably not working to remove carbon dioxide from the body quickly, blood pH levels drop. This will happen more often if a person has a chronic or severe lung condition, such as:

- Diaphragm disorders
- Chronic obstructive pulmonary disease
- Pneumonia
- Bronchitis

- Sleep apnea
- Asthma

People who are obese, have had surgery, or abuse opioid painkillers or sedatives are at increased risk of developing respiratory acidosis. In some cases, the kidneys can take over the situation and remove excess blood acids through excretion. As a result, a person may need to receive extra oxygen and medications such as steroids and bronchodilators to help the lungs function correctly. In very severe cases, mechanical ventilation and intubation may be needed in individuals with respiratory acidosis to bring the blood pH back to normal.

- Urine pH

The next type of pH we will examine is urine pH. Urine is composed of waste products, salts, and water that are excreted through the kidneys. The balance of these different compounds can affect the acidity level of the urine. According to the American Association for Clinical Chemistry, the average urine pH is 6.0, but it can range from 4.5 to 8.0. Any level below 5.0 is considered acidic urine, and any level above 8.0 is considered basic urine.

Sometimes different labs have different ranges on what they consider normal pH levels for urine. One of the main things that affect the pH of your urine is the things you eat. If you go to your doctor, he or she will often ask you what foods you ate before evaluating the results of a urine pH test.

If, before a test, you ate more acidic foods, your urine will be more acidic. The same is true if you have eaten more alkaline foods. If a person has extremely high pH levels in their urine, meaning it is more alkaline, it could be the result of problems, such as:

- Urinary tract infections
- Kidney stones
- Other kidney-related disorders

A person may also have high pH levels in their urine if they have had prolonged vomiting. This is because vomiting causes the body to get rid of stomach acid, which causes body fluids to become more essential.

When urine is acidic, it creates an environment conducive to kidney stones. When urine is acidic, it can also be a sign of several severe medical conditions, such as:

- Hunger
- Diarrhea
- Diabetic ketoacidosis

As you will notice, much of this is the same as blood pH levels. Certain medications can affect the pH of the urine. Sometimes doctors will ask a patient to discontinue certain medications the day or night before doing a urinalysis.

- Saliva pH

The last pH we will look at is the pH of saliva. The usual range of saliva pH is from 6.2 to 7.6. The things you drink and eat can change the pH of your saliva.

Just like any other area of your body, your mouth needs to maintain a balanced pH. Saliva pH levels can drop below 5.5 when you've had a lot of acidic drinks. When this happens, the acids in your mouth begin to break down the enamel on your teeth.

If your tooth enamel becomes too thin, the dentin will be exposed. This can end up causing discomfort when you consume sugary, cold, or hot drinks. Just to give you an example of foods and drinks that can do this, here are some numbers:

- Cherries have a pH of 4
- American cheese has a pH of 5
- White wine has a pH of 4
- Soft drinks have a pH of 3

It's easy to spot unbalanced pH levels in your saliva. Some of the most common indicators are:
- Tooth decay
- Sensitivity to cold or hot drinks or foods
- Persistent bad breath

If you want, you can also test the pH of your saliva. Your saliva's pH can be tested: you will need to find pH strips. Once you have your strips, this is what you need to do:
- Make sure you don't eat or drink anything for at least two hours before the test.
- Let your mouth fill with saliva and then swallow or spit it out.
- Let your mouth fill with saliva again, and then place a small amount on one of your pH strips.
- The strip will then react to your saliva. It will change color based on how alkaline or acidic your saliva is. The container the pH strips came with should show a color chart. Put your strip next to the chart to match the colors and determine the pH level of your saliva.

To make sure the pH of your saliva stays balanced, you must eat foods that are in a healthy pH range. It's also important that you don't deprive yourself of important vitamins and minerals. There are a few more effective ways to make sure the pH of your saliva stays balanced.
- Stay away from sugary drinks. If you must drink them, try to drink them quickly and chase them with water. Sipping sugary beverages for an extended period of time does more damage.
- Limit black coffee. Adding a little cream, unsweetened, can help reduce the acidity of coffee.
- Avoid brushing your teeth immediately after consuming high-acid beverages such as beer, wine, cider, juice, or soda. These types of beverages soften tooth enamel. If you brush your teeth too soon after consuming these things, you will further damage your enamel.
- Chew sugar-free gum after consuming any beverage or food. Chewing gum will cause your mouth to produce more saliva and help bring your pH level back to normal. It is also believed that xylitol can prevent bacteria from sticking to your tooth enamel.
- Keep yourself hydrated, so be sure to drink plenty of water.

BREAKFAST & SMOOTHIES

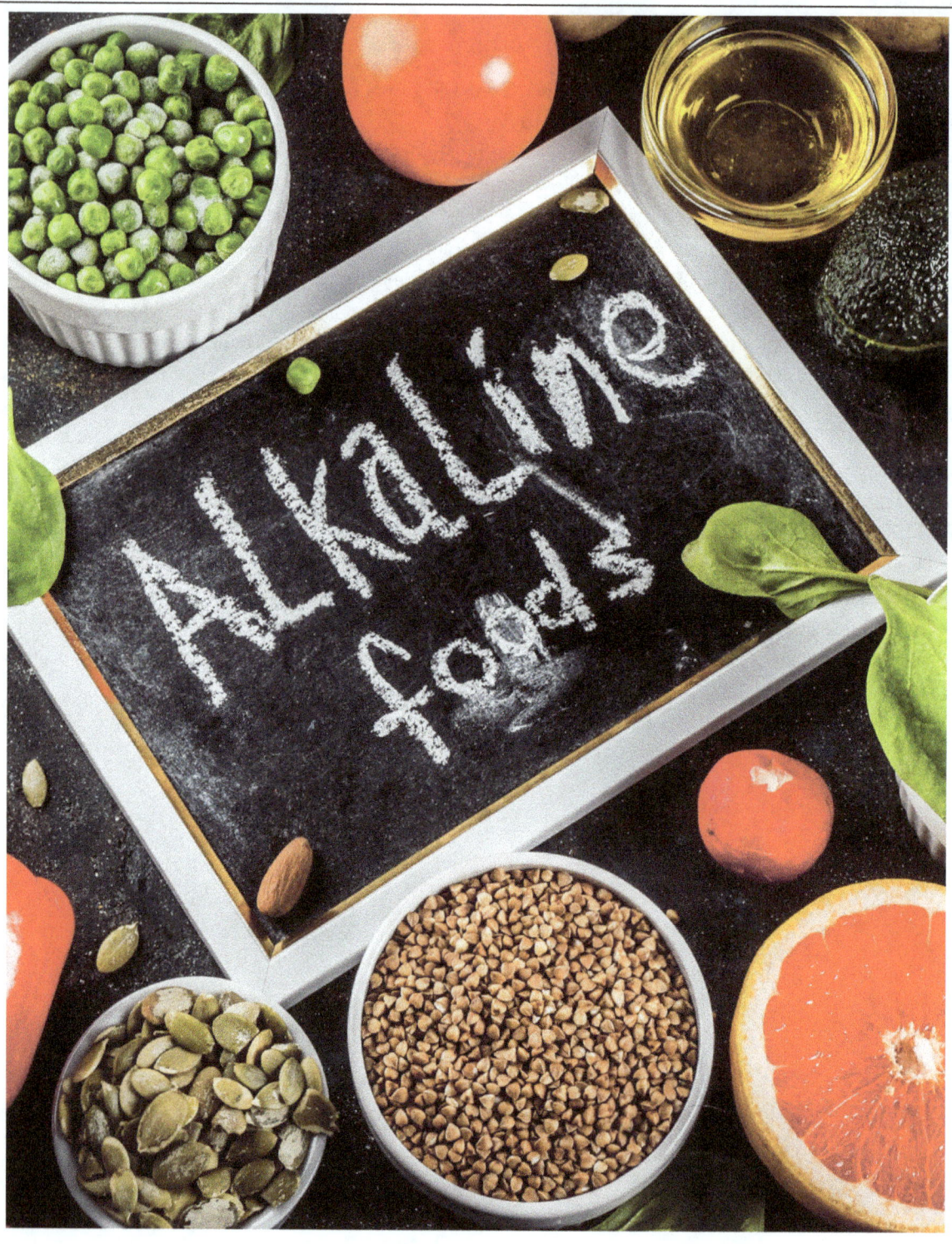

109) Chocolate quinoa porridge

Preparation time: 15 minutes **Cooking time:** 30 minutes **Portions: 4**

Ingredients:
- 1 cup uncooked quinoa, rinsed and drained
- 1 cup unsweetened almond milk
- 1 cup unsweetened coconut milk
- Pinch of sea salt

Directions:
- Heat a small non-stick frying pan over medium heat and cook the quinoa for about 3 minutes or until lightly toasted, stirring often.
- Add the almond milk, coconut milk and a pinch of salt and stir to combine.
- Increase the heat to high and bring to the boil.

Ingredients:
- 2 tablespoons of cocoa powder
- 2 tablespoons maple syrup
- ½ teaspoon organic vanilla extract
- ½ cup fresh strawberries, peeled and sliced

- Reduce the heat to low and cook, uncovered for about 20-25 minutes or until all the liquid is absorbed, stirring occasionally.
- Remove from the heat and immediately stir in the cocoa powder, maple syrup and vanilla extract.
- Serve immediately with a garnish of strawberry slices.

110) Buckwheat porridge with walnuts

Preparation time: 15 minutes **Cooking time:** 7 minutes **Portions: 2**

Ingredients:
- ½ cup buckwheat
- 1 cup of alkaline water
- 2 tablespoons of chia seeds
- 15-20 almonds
- 1 cup unsweetened almond milk

Directions:
- In a large bowl, soak the buckwheat groats in water overnight.
- In 2 other bowls, soak the chia seeds and almonds respectively.
- Drain the buckwheat and rinse well.
- In a non-stick pan, add the buckwheat and almond milk over medium heat and cook for about 7 minutes or until creamy.

Ingredients:
- ½ teaspoon cinnamon powder
- 1 teaspoon organic vanilla extract
- 3-4 drops of liquid stevia
- ¼ cup of fresh mixed berries

- Drain the chia seeds and almonds well.
- Remove the pan from the heat and stir in the almonds, chia seeds, cinnamon, vanilla extract and stevia.
- Serve hot with a berry garnish.

111) Fruity oatmeal

Preparation time: 15 minutes
Cooking time: 10 minutes
Portions: 4

Ingredients:
- 4 cups of alkaline water
- 1 cup steel-cut dry oats
- 1 large banana, peeled and mashed

Ingredients:
- 1½ cups of fresh mixed berries (your choice)
- ¼ cup walnuts, finely chopped

Directions:
- In a large pan, add the water and oats over medium-high heat and bring to the boil.
- Reduce the heat to low and simmer for about 20 minutes, stirring occasionally.
- Remove from the heat and cool slightly.
- Add the mashed banana and stir to combine.
- Cover with strawberries and walnuts and serve.

112) Baked walnut oatmeal

Preparation time: 15 minutes
Cooking time: 45 minutes
Portions: 5

Ingredients:
- 1 tablespoon linseed meal
- 3 tablespoons of alkaline water
- 3 cups unsweetened almond milk
- ¼ cup maple syrup
- 2 tablespoons coconut oil, melted and cooled
- 2 teaspoons of organic vanilla extract

Ingredients:
- 1 teaspoon cinnamon powder
- 1 teaspoon organic baking powder
- ¼ teaspoon of sea salt
- 2 cups old rolled oats
- ½ cup almonds, chopped
- ½ cup walnuts, chopped

Directions:
- Lightly grease an 8x8-inch baking dish. Set aside.
- In a large bowl, add the flaxseed meal and water and beat until well combined. Set aside for about 5 minutes.
- In the bowl of the flax mixture, add the remaining ingredients except the oats and nuts and mix until well combined.
- Add the oats and nuts and stir gently to combine.
- Place the mixture in the prepared baking tin and spread it out in an even layer.
- Cover the baking tray with plastic wrap and refrigerate for about 8 hours.
- Preheat the oven to 350 degrees F. Place a wire rack in the centre of the oven.
- Remove the tray from the refrigerator and let it rest at room temperature for 15-20 minutes.
- Remove the plastic film and mix the oatmeal mixture well.
- Bake for about 45 minutes.
- Remove from the oven and set aside to cool slightly.
- Serve hot.

113) Almond fritters

Preparation time:
Cooking time:
Portions: 4

Ingredients:
- Coconut oil, 3 tablespoons
- Almond milk, 1 c.
- Baking powder, 1 teaspoon

Ingredients:
- Arrowroot powder, 2 tablespoons
- Almond flour, 1 c.

Directions:
- Place each of the dry fixings in a dish and whisk to mix.
- Add two tablespoons of coconut oil together with the almond milk to the dry elements and mix well until everything is combined.
- Place a frying pan over medium heat and put a teaspoon of coconut to melt. Swirl it around in the pan to coat it.
- Pour a ladleful of batter into the pan and use the bottom of the ladle to smooth out the pancake.
- Bake for three minutes until the edges are bubbly and brown.
- Flip the pancake over and cook for a further three minutes until cooked through.
- Continue to cook the pancakes until all the batter has been used.

114) Amaranth porridge

Preparation time: **Cooking time**: **Portions: 2**

Ingredients:
- ✓ Cinnamon, 1 tablespoon
- ✓ Coconut oil, 2 tablespoons
- ✓ Amaranth, 1 c.

Ingredients:
- ✓ Alkaline water, 2 c.
- ✓ Almond milk, 2 c.

Directions:
- ❖ Put the water and milk in a saucepan. Set to medium-hot and let it boil.
- ❖ Add the amaranth and lower the heat to low. Stew for half an hour, stirring occasionally.
- ❖ Remove from the heat, add the copra oil and cinnamon, mix well, serve hot.

115) Banana porridge

Preparation time: **Cooking time**: **Portions: 2**

Ingredients:
- ✓ Ground almonds, .25 c.
- ✓ Liquid stevia, 3 drops
- ✓ Barley, .5 c.

Ingredients:
- ✓ Sliced banana, 1
- ✓ Unsweetened almond milk, 1 c.

Directions:
- ❖ Mix stevia, 1/2 cup almond milk and barley in a bowl.
- ❖ Refrigerate, covered for six hours.
- ❖ Remove from the fridge and mix with the remaining milk. Pour into a saucepan and place on medium. Allow the mixture to cook for five minutes.

116) Courgette muffins

Preparation time: **Cooking time**: **Portions: 16**

Ingredients:
- ✓ Halls
- ✓ Cinnamon, 1 teaspoon
- ✓ Baking powder, 1 tablespoon
- ✓ Almond flour, 2 c.
- ✓ Vanilla extract, 1 teaspoon
- ✓ Almond milk, .5 c.
- ✓ Grated courgettes, 2

Ingredients:
- ✓ Overripe bananas, 3
- ✓ Almond butter, .25 c.
- ✓ Alkaline water, 3 tablespoons
- ✓ Ground linseed, 1 tablespoon
- ✓ Optional ingredients:
- ✓ Chopped walnuts, .25 c.
- ✓ Chocolate chips, .25 c.

Directions:
- ❖ You need to heat your cooking appliance to 375 degrees. Spray a cupcake pan with cooking spray.
- ❖ Place the water and linseed in a bowl.
- ❖ Mash the bananas in a saucepan and put all the leftover contents in. Stir well.
- ❖ Spread the concoction evenly in a cupcake tin.
- ❖ Bake for 25 minutes.

117) Tofu stew with vegetables

Preparation time: **Cooking time**: **Portions: 4**

Ingredients:
- ✓ Halls
- ✓ Chopped basil, 2 tablespoons
- ✓ Chopped hard-boiled tofu, 3 c.
- ✓ Diced peppers (red, bell), 2 pieces.
- ✓ Olive oil, 1 tablespoon

Ingredients:
- ✓ Turmeric
- ✓ Chopped cherry tomatoes, 2 c.
- ✓ Chopped onions, 2
- ✓ Cayenne

Directions:
- ❖ Place a greased frying pan over medium heat and heat the pan.
- ❖ Put the peppers together with the onions, prepare for five minutes.
- ❖ Add the tofu, cayenne, salt and turmeric. Cook for a further eight minutes.
- ❖ Garnish with basil.

118) Courgette fritters

Preparation time: **Cooking time:** **Portions:** 8

Ingredients:
- ✓ Shallots, finely chopped, .5 c.
- ✓ Finely chopped jalapeno, 2
- ✓ Olive oil, 2 tablespoons
- ✓ Ground linseed, 4 tablespoons

Directions:
- ❖ Place the flaxseed and water in a bowl and mix well. Set aside.
- ❖ Place a large frying pan over medium heat and heat the oil. Add the pepper, salt and courgettes. Cook for three minutes and place the courgettes in a bowl.

Ingredients:
- ✓ Halls
- ✓ Grated courgettes, 6
- ✓ Alkaline water, 12 tablespoons

- ❖ Add the linseed mixture and the shallots and mix well.
- ❖ Heat up a griddle that has been sprayed with cooking spray. Pour a few courgettes onto the preheated griddle and cook for three minutes per side until golden brown.
- ❖ Repeat until the mixture is completely exhausted.

119) Quinoa with pumpkin

Preparation time: **Cooking time:** **Portions:** 2

Ingredients:
- ✓ Chia seeds, 2 teaspoons
- ✓ Pumpkin pie spice, 1 teaspoon
- ✓ Pumpkin puree, .25 c.

Directions:
- ❖ Put all the ingredients in a container.
- ❖ Make sure the lid is sealed and shake well to combine.

Ingredients:
- ✓ Crushed banana, 1
- ✓ Unsweetened almond milk, 1 c.
- ✓ Cooked quinoa, 1 c.
- ❖ Refrigerate overnight.
- ❖ When ready to eat, take it out of the fridge and enjoy.

120) Avocado toast

Preparation time: **Cooking time:** **Portions:** 4

Ingredients:
- ✓ Dulse flakes, sliced radish, sliced red onion, for garnish - optional
- ✓ Sea salt, 0.5 teaspoons
- ✓ Fresh coriander leaves, 1 tablespoon
- ✓ Chopped onion, 1 tablespoon

Directions:
- ❖ Place each of the potato slices in a slot of the toaster and toast them for four cycles, or until they are cooked. You can also toast them in the oven if you don't have a regular toaster oven. You want them to be tender enough that you can easily pierce them with a fork. Carefully arrange the cooked toast on plates.

Ingredients:
- ✓ Garlic, 2 cloves
- ✓ Jalapeno
- ✓ Avocado, 2
- ✓ Sweet potato, unpeeled, cut into 4 thick slices lengthwise
- ❖ While the sweet potato toast is cooking, add the salt, coriander, onion, garlic, jalapeno and avocado to an extremely electric food processor and blend until smooth. Adjust the amount of salt as necessary.
- ❖ Divide the avocado spread over each of the sweet potato toast slices. Top each slice with the desired toppings. Enjoy your meal.

121) Frozen banana breakfast bowl

Preparation time: **Cooking time:** **Portions:** 1

Ingredients:
- ✓ Chia seeds, hemp seeds, unsweetened coconut flakes, for garnish - optional
- ✓ Pumpkin seed protein powder, 4 tablespoons

Directions:
- ❖ Peel and then slice the bananas. Place them thinly in a freezer-safe container and freeze overnight.
- ❖ The next morning, add the bananas to a food processor and blend until a smooth, creamy consistency is achieved, much like that of soft-serve ice cream.

Ingredients:
- ✓ Bananas, 2

- ❖ Process the pumpkin protein powder through the bananas until it is just combined.
- ❖ Pour into a serving dish and add the desired toppings, if desired, and enjoy.

LUNCH

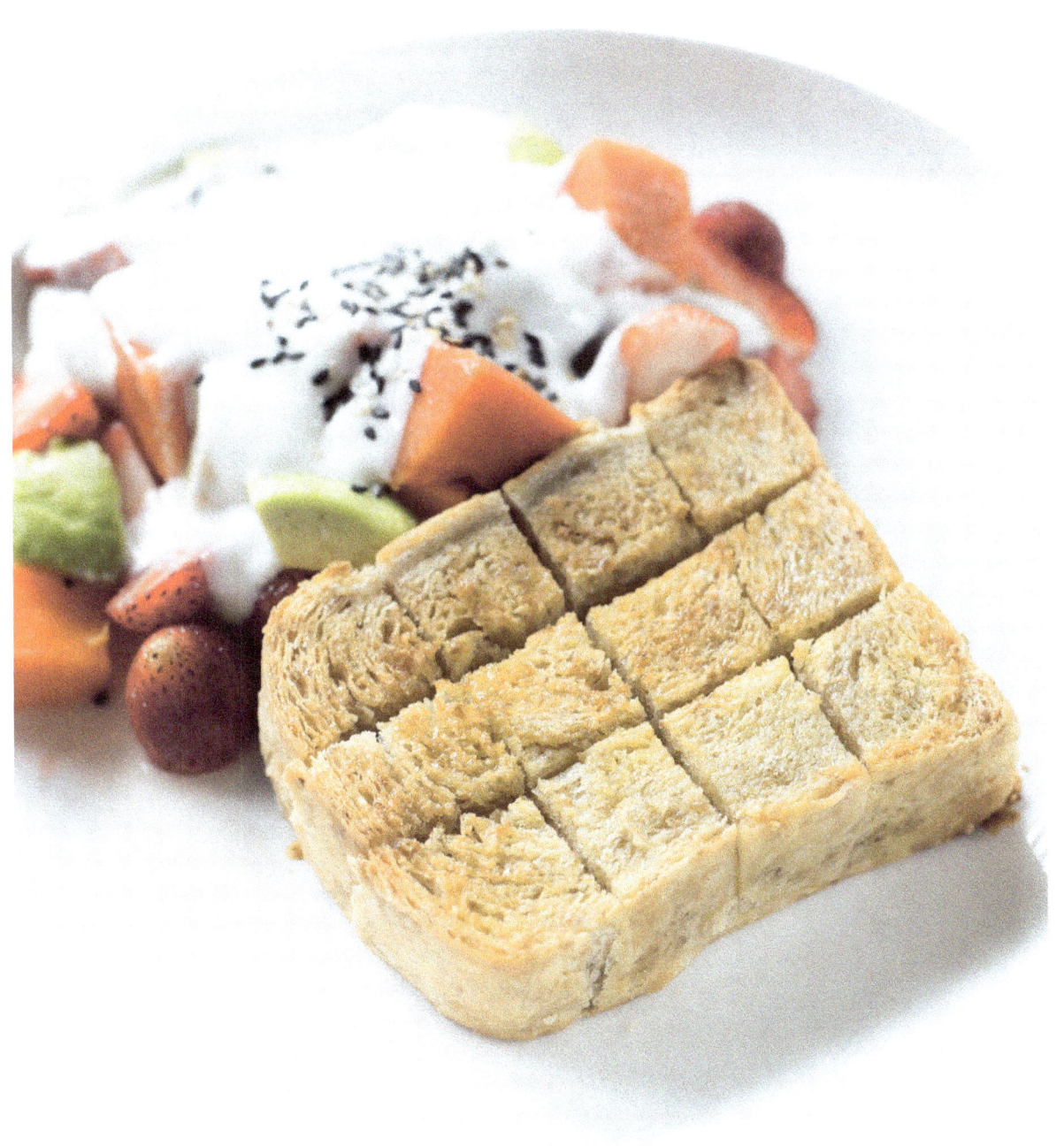

122) Vegetarian lettuce rolls

Preparation time: 20 minutes **Cooking time**: 10 minutes **Portions**: 4

Ingredients:
- For filling:
- 1 teaspoon of olive oil
- 2 cups fresh shiitake mushrooms, chopped
- 2 teaspoons of tamari, divided
- 1 cup of cooked quinoa
- 1 teaspoon fresh lime juice
- 1 teaspoon organic apple cider vinegar
- ¼ cup shallots, chopped
- Sea salt and freshly ground black pepper, to taste
- For the creamy sauce:
- 5 ounces of tofu silken, pressed, drained and chopped
- 1 small clove of garlic, minced

Ingredients:
- ¼ cup plain almond butter
- 1 teaspoon fresh lime juice
- Sea salt and freshly ground black pepper, to taste
- For enclosures:
- 8 medium-sized lettuce leaves
- ¼ cup cucumber, peeled and julienned
- ¼ cup of carrot, peeled and julienned
- ¼ cup of cabbage, shredded

Directions:
- For the filling, in a frying pan, heat the oil over medium heat and cook the mushrooms and 1 teaspoon of tamari for about 5-8 minutes, stirring often.
- Stir in the quinoa, lime juice, vinegar and remaining tamari and cook for about 1 minute, stirring constantly.
- Add the shallot, salt and black pepper and immediately remove from the heat.
- Set aside to cool.
- Meanwhile, for the sauce: in a food processor, add all the ingredients and pulse until a smooth sauce is obtained.
- Arrange the lettuce leaves on serving plates.
- Place the quinoa filling evenly on each leaf and cover with cucumbers, carrots and cabbage.
- Serve alongside the creamy sauce.

123) Oatmeal, tofu and spinach burger

Preparation time: 15 minutes **Cooking time**: 16 minutes **Portions**: 4

Ingredients:
- 1 pound firm tofu, drained, pressed and crumbled
- ¾ cup rolled oats
- ¼ cup of linseed
- 2 cups of frozen, thawed, squeezed and chopped cabbage
- 1 medium onion, finely chopped
- 4 cloves of garlic, minced

Ingredients:
- 1 teaspoon ground cumin
- 1 teaspoon red pepper flakes, crushed
- Sea salt and freshly ground black pepper, to taste
- 2 tablespoons of olive oil
- 6 cups of fresh salad

Directions:
- In a large bowl, add all the ingredients except the oil and the green salads and mix until well combined.
- Set aside for about 10 minutes.
- Cut the dough into meatballs of the desired size.
- In a non-stick frying pan, heat the oil over medium heat and cook the meatballs for 6-8 minutes per side.
- Serve these meatballs alongside green salad.

124) Hamburger with beans, nuts and vegetables

Preparation time: 20 minutes **Cooking time**: 25 minutes **Portions**: 4

Ingredients:
- ½ cup walnuts
- 1 carrot, peeled and chopped
- 1 celery stalk, chopped
- 4 shallots, chopped
- 5 cloves of garlic, minced
- 2¼ cups canned black beans, rinsed and drained

Directions:
- Preheat the oven to 400 degrees F. Line a baking tray with baking paper.
- In a food processor, add the walnuts and pulse until finely ground.
- Add the carrot, celery, shallot and garlic and chop finely.
- Transfer the vegetable mixture into a large bowl.
- In the same food processor, add the beans and give a pulse until they are chopped.
- Add 1 1/2 cups of sweet potatoes and pulse to form a chunky mixture.

Ingredients:
- 2½ cups sweet potato, peeled and grated
- ½ teaspoon red pepper flakes, crushed
- ¼ teaspoon cayenne pepper
- Sea salt and freshly ground black pepper, to taste
- 12 cups of fresh vegetables

- Transfer the bean mixture to the bowl with the vegetable mixture.
- Stir in the remaining sweet potato, spices, salt and black pepper and mix until well combined.
- Make 8 equal-sized patties from the bean mixture.
- Arrange the meatballs on the prepared baking tray in a single layer.
- Bake for about 25 minutes.
- Divide the vegetables between the serving plates and top each with 2 meatballs.
- Serve immediately.

125) Avocado stuffed with tofu and broccoli

Preparation time: 20 minutes **Cooking time**: 15 minutes **Portions**: 6

Ingredients:
  For the marinade:
- ¼ cup fresh parsley leaves, chopped
- 1 small clove of garlic, minced
- 1 teaspoon fresh lemon peel, finely grated
- 1 tablespoon Dijon mustard
- ¼ cup of olive oil
- 2 tablespoons fresh lemon juice
- ¼ teaspoon of ground cumin
- Sea salt and freshly ground black pepper, to taste

Directions:
- For the marinade: in a large bowl, add all the ingredients except the tofu and beat until well combined.
- Add the tofu and broccoli and cover generously with the marinade.
- Cover the bowl and refrigerate for about 1 hour.
- Preheat the grill to medium-high heat. Generously grease the grill grate.
- Place the tofu slices on the grill and cook for about 2 minutes per side.
- Grill the broccoli florets for about 8-10 minutes, turning occasionally.

Ingredients:
- 1 (8-ounce) package of solid tofu, drained, pressed and cut into ½ inch slices
- 1 cup of broccoli florets
  For the stuffed avocados:
- 1 tablespoon fresh chives, chopped
- 3 firm avocados, peeled, halved and pitted
- Sea salt and freshly ground black pepper, to taste
- 2 tablespoons fresh parsley, chopped

- Remove the tofu and broccoli from the grill and transfer to a large bowl.
- Set aside to cool slightly.
- Then, cut the tofu and broccoli into small pieces.
- Transfer the tofu and broccoli to a bowl with the chives and mix well.
- Sprinkle the avocado halves with salt and black pepper.
- Stuff each half evenly with the tofu mixture.
- Garnish with parsley and serve immediately.

126) Brussels sprouts with walnuts

Preparation time: 15 minutes **Cooking time**: 15 minutes **Portions**: 2

Ingredients:
- ½ pound Brussels sprouts, cut and halved
- 1 tablespoon olive oil
- 2 cloves of garlic, minced
- ½ teaspoon red pepper flakes, crushed

Directions:
- In a large pot of boiling water, place a steamer basket.
- Place the asparagus in the basket of the steamer and steam, covered, for about 6-8 minutes.
- Drain the asparagus well.

Ingredients:
- Sea salt and freshly ground black pepper, to taste
- 1 tablespoon fresh lemon juice
- 1 tablespoon pine nuts

- In a large frying pan, heat the oil over medium heat and fry the garlic and red pepper flakes for about 30-40 seconds.
- Add the Brussels sprouts, salt and black pepper and fry for about 4-5 minutes.
- Add the lemon juice and fry for about 1 minute more.
- Add the pine nuts and remove from the heat.
- Serve hot.

127) Broccoli with cabbage

Preparation time: 20 minutes **Cooking time**: 1 hour 20 minutes **Portions**: 8

Ingredients:
- 3 tablespoons of coconut oil, divided by
- ¼ small yellow onion, chopped
- 1 teaspoon chopped garlic
- 1 teaspoon fresh ginger root, peeled and chopped
- 1 cup of broccoli florets

Directions:
- In a large frying pan, melt 2 tablespoons of coconut oil over medium-high heat and fry the onion for about 3-4 minutes.
- Add the garlic and ginger and fry for about 1 minute.
- Add the broccoli and stir to combine well.
- Immediately, reduce the heat to medium-low and cook for about 2-3 minutes, stirring constantly.

Ingredients:
- 2 cups fresh cabbage, hard ribs removed and chopped
- ½ cup of coconut cream
- ¼ teaspoon red pepper flakes, crushed
- 1 teaspoon fresh parsley, finely chopped

- Add the cabbage and cook for about 3 minutes, stirring often.
- Add the coconut cream and the remaining coconut oil and mix until smooth.
- Add the red pepper flakes and simmer for about 5-10 minutes, stirring occasionally or until the curry has the desired thickness.
- Remove from the heat and serve hot with a garnish of parsley.

128) Mushrooms with parsley

Preparation time: 15 minutes **Cooking time**: 15 minutes **Portions**: 2

Ingredients:
- 2 tablespoons of olive oil
- 2-3 tablespoons of chopped onion
- ½ teaspoon chopped garlic

Directions:
- In a frying pan, heat the oil over medium heat and fry the onion and garlic for 2-3 minutes.

Ingredients:
- 12 ounces of sliced fresh mushrooms
- 1 tablespoon fresh parsley, chopped
- Sea salt and freshly ground black pepper, to taste

- Add the mushrooms and cook for 8-10 minutes or until cooked through, stirring frequently.
- Add the parsley, salt and black pepper and remove from the heat.
- Serve hot.

129) Garlic broccoli

Preparation time: 15 minutes   **Cooking time:** 8 minutes   **Portions: 3**

Ingredients:
- 1 tablespoon olive oil
- 2 cloves of garlic, minced
- 2 cups of broccoli florets

Directions:
- In a large frying pan, heat the oil over medium heat and fry the garlic for about 1 minute.
- Add the broccoli and fry for about 2 minutes.

Ingredients:
- 2 tablespoons of alkaline water
- Sea salt and freshly ground black pepper, to taste

- In a large frying pan, heat the oil over medium heat and fry the garlic for about 1 minute.
- Add the broccoli and fry for about 2 minutes.

130) Broccoli with peppers

Preparation time: 15 minutes   **Cooking time:** 10 minutes   **Portions: 5**

Ingredients:
- 2 tablespoons of olive oil
- 4 cloves of garlic, minced
- 1 large white onion, sliced
- 2 cups of small broccoli florets

Directions:
- In a large frying pan, heat the oil over medium heat and fry the garlic for about 1 minute.

Ingredients:
- 3 red peppers, seeded and sliced
- ¼ cup of homemade vegetable stock
- Sea salt and freshly ground black pepper, to taste

- Add the onion, broccoli and peppers and fry for about 5 minutes.
- Add the stock and fry for about 4 minutes more.
- Serve hot.

131) Spicy okra

Preparation time: 15 minutes   **Cooking time:** 13 minutes   **Portions: 2**

Ingredients:
- 1 tablespoon olive oil
- ½ teaspoon of caraway seeds
- ¾ pound okra pods, trimmed and cut into 2-inch pieces

Directions:
- In a large frying pan, heat the oil over medium heat and fry the cumin seeds for 30 seconds.
- Add the okra and fry for 1-1½ minutes.
- Reduce the heat to low and cook, covered, for 6-8 minutes, stirring occasionally.

Ingredients:
- ½ teaspoon of red chilli powder
- 1 teaspoon ground coriander
- Sea salt and freshly ground black pepper, to taste

- Uncover and increase heat to medium.
- Add the chilli powder and cilantro and cook for a further 2-3 minutes.
- Season with salt and remove from the heat.
- Serve hot.

132) Spicy cauliflower

Preparation time: 15 minutes **Cooking time**: 20 minutes **Portions**: 4

Ingredients:
- ¼ cup alkaline water
- 2 medium fresh tomatoes, chopped
- 2 tablespoons of extra virgin olive oil
- 1 small white onion, chopped
- ½ tablespoon fresh ginger root, peeled and chopped
- 3 medium garlic cloves, chopped
- 1 jalapeño pepper, seeded and chopped
- 1 teaspoon ground cumin

Ingredients:
- 1 teaspoon ground coriander
- 1 teaspoon cayenne pepper
- ¼ teaspoon ground turmeric
- 3 cups cauliflower, chopped
- Sea salt and freshly ground black pepper, to taste
- ½ cup of warm alkaline water
- ¼ cup fresh parsley leaves, chopped

Directions:
- In a blender, add ¼ cup water and the tomatoes and pulse until pureed. Set aside.
- In a large frying pan, heat the oil over medium heat and fry the onion for about 4-5 minutes.
- Add the ginger, garlic, jalapeño pepper and spices and fry for about 1 minute.
- Add the tomato puree and cauliflower and cook for about 3-4 minutes, stirring constantly.
- Add the hot water and bring to the boil.
- Reduce the heat to medium-low and simmer, covered, for about 8-10 minutes or until the desired doneness of the cauliflower.
- Remove from the heat and serve hot with a garnish of parsley.

133) Aubergine curry

Preparation time: 15 minutes **Cooking time**: 35 minutes **Portions**: 3

Ingredients:
- 1 tablespoon of coconut oil
- 1 medium onion, finely chopped
- 2 cloves of garlic, minced
- ½ tablespoon fresh ginger root, peeled and chopped
- 1 Serrano pepper, seeded and chopped

Ingredients:
- Sea salt and freshly ground black pepper, to taste
- 1 medium tomato, finely chopped
- 1 large aubergine, diced
- 1 cup unsweetened coconut milk
- 2 tablespoons fresh parsley, chopped

Directions:
- In a large frying pan, melt the coconut oil over medium heat and fry the onion for 8-9 minutes.
- Add the garlic, serrano pepper and salt and fry for 1 minute.
- Add the tomato and cook for 3-4 minutes, crushing with the back of a spoon.
- Add the aubergines and salt and cook for 1 minute, stirring occasionally.
- Stir in the coconut milk and bring to a gentle boil.
- Reduce the heat to medium-low and simmer, covered for 15-20 minutes or until completely done.
- Remove from the heat and serve with a garnish of parsley.

134) Lemon cabbage with shallots

Preparation time: 15 minutes **Cooking time**: 20 minutes **Portions**: 4

Ingredients:
- 1 tablespoon extra virgin olive oil
- 1 lemon, seeded and thinly sliced
- 1 white onion, thinly sliced
- 3 cloves of garlic, minced

Ingredients:
- 2 lbs. fresh cabbage, hard ribs removed and chopped
- ½ cup shallots, chopped
- Sea salt and freshly ground black pepper, to taste

Directions:
- In a large frying pan, heat the oil over medium heat and cook the lemon slices for 5 minutes.
- Using a slotted spoon, remove the lemon slices from the pan and set aside.
- In the same pan, add the onion and garlic and fry for about 5 minutes.
- Add the cabbage, shallots, salt and pepper and cook for 8-10 minutes.
- Add the lemon slices and stir until well combined.
- Remove from the heat and serve hot.

135) Vegetables with apple

Preparation time: 15 minutes **Cooking time**: 16 minutes **Portions**: 4

Ingredients:

For the sauce:
- 3 small garlic cloves, chopped
- 1 teaspoon fresh ginger root, peeled and chopped
- 1 tablespoon fresh orange peel, finely grated
- ½ cup of fresh orange juice
- 1 tablespoon maple syrup
- 2 tablespoons of tamari
- 2 tablespoons organic apple cider vinegar

Directions:
- For the sauce: in a large bowl, add all the ingredients and with a wire whisk, beat until well combined. Set aside.
- In a large frying pan, heat the oil over medium-high heat and fry the carrot and broccoli for about 4-5 minutes.

Ingredients:

For vegetables and apple:
- 1 tablespoon olive oil
- 2 cups of carrots, peeled and cut into julienne strips
- 1 head of broccoli, cut into florets
- 1 cup red onion, chopped
- 2 apples, core and slices

- Add the onion and fry for about 4-5 minutes.
- Add the sauce and cook for about 2-3 minutes, stirring frequently.
- Stir in the apple slices and cook for about 2-3 minutes.
- Remove from the heat and serve hot.

136) Cabbage with apple

Preparation time: 15 minutes **Cooking time:** 12 minutes **Portions:** 4

Ingredients:
- 2 teaspoons of coconut oil
- 1 large apple, cored and thinly sliced
- 1 onion, thinly sliced
- 1 ½ pounds of cabbage, finely chopped

Directions:
- In a non-stick pan, melt 1 teaspoon of coconut oil over medium heat and fry the apple for about 2-3 minutes.
- Transfer the apple to a bowl.
- In the same pan, melt 1 teaspoon of coconut oil over medium heat and fry the onion for about 2-3 minutes.

Ingredients:
- 1 tablespoon fresh thyme, chopped
- 1 fresh red chilli pepper, chopped
- 1 tablespoon organic apple cider vinegar

- Add the cabbage and fry for about 4-5 minutes.
- Add the cooked apple slices, thyme and vinegar and cook, covered, for about 1 minute.
- Remove from the heat and serve hot.

137) Asparagus with herbs

Preparation time: 15 minutes **Cooking time:** 10 minutes **Portions:** 4

Ingredients:
- 2 tablespoons of olive oil
- 2 tablespoons fresh lemon juice
- 1 tablespoon organic apple cider vinegar
- 1 teaspoon chopped garlic

Directions:
- Preheat the oven to 400 degrees F. Lightly grease a rimmed baking sheet.
- In a bowl, add the oil, lemon juice, vinegar, garlic, herbs, salt and black pepper and whisk until well combined.

Ingredients:
- 1 tablespoon fresh parsley, chopped
- 1 teaspoon dried oregano
- Sea salt and freshly ground black pepper, to taste
- 1 lb. fresh asparagus, without ends
- Arrange the asparagus on the prepared baking tray in a single layer.
- Cover with half of the herb mixture and stir to coat.
- Roast for about 8-10 minutes.
- Remove from the oven and transfer the asparagus to a serving dish.
- Sprinkle with the remaining herb mixture and serve immediately.

138) Vegetarian Kabobs

Preparation time: 20 minutes **Cooking time:** 10 minutes **Portions:** 4

Ingredients:

For the marinade:
- 2 cloves of garlic, minced
- 2 teaspoons fresh basil, chopped
- 2 teaspoons fresh oregano, chopped
- ½ teaspoon of cayenne pepper
- Sea salt and freshly ground black pepper, to taste
- 2 tablespoons fresh lemon juice
- 2 tablespoons of olive oil

Directions:
- For the marinade: in a large bowl, add all the ingredients and mix until well combined.
- Add the vegetables and toss to coat them well.
- Cover the bowl and place in the fridge to marinate for at least 6-8 hours.
- Preheat the grill to medium-high heat. Generously grease the grill grate.

Ingredients:

For the vegetables:
- 16 large button mushrooms, quartered
- 1 yellow pepper, seeded and diced
- 1 red pepper, seeded and diced
- 1 orange pepper, seeded and diced
- 1 green pepper, seeded and diced

- Remove the vegetables from the bowl and thread onto pre-soaked wooden skewers.
- Place the skewers on the grill and cook for about 8-10 minutes or until cooked through, turning occasionally.
- Remove from the grill and serve hot.

139) Tofu with Brussels sprouts

Preparation time: 15 minutes **Cooking time:** 15 minutes **Portions:** 4

Ingredients:
- 1 tablespoon olive oil, separated
- 8 ounces of extra-fine tofu, drained, pressed and sliced
- 2 cloves of garlic, minced
- 1/3 cup pecans, toasted and chopped

Directions:
- In a frying pan, heat ½ tablespoon of oil over medium heat and fry the tofu for about 6-7 minutes or until golden brown.
- Add the garlic and pecans and fry for about 1 minute.
- Add the apple sauce and cook for about 2 minutes.
- Add the parsley and remove from the heat.

Ingredients:
- 1 tablespoon unsweetened apple juice
- ¼ cup fresh parsley, chopped
- ½ pound Brussels sprouts, trimmed and cut into wide strips

- With a slotted spoon, transfer the tofu to a plate and set aside.
- In the same pan, heat the remaining oil over medium-high heat and cook the Brussels sprouts for about 5 minutes.
- Stir in the cooked tofu and remove from the heat.
- Serve immediately.

140) Tofu with broccoli

Preparation time: 15 minutes **Cooking time:** 13 minutes **Portions:** 3

Ingredients:
- 1 (12-ounce) package of solid tofu, drained, pressed and cut into 5 slices
- 2 tablespoons of coconut oil, divided by
- 2 cups of small broccoli florets

Directions:
- In a large non-stick frying pan, melt 1 tablespoon of coconut oil over medium-high heat and cook the tofu for 4-5 minutes per side or until crispy.
- Using a slotted spoon, place the tofu slices on a paper towel-lined plate to absorb the extra oil.
- Then, cut each slice of tofu into equal-sized pieces.
- Meanwhile, in a large microwaveable bowl, add the broccoli florets and water.

Ingredients:
- ¼ cup alkaline water
- ½ tablespoon chopped garlic
- ½ tablespoon fresh ginger root, chopped
- Sea salt and freshly ground black pepper, to taste

- Cover the bowl and microwave on High for about 5 minutes.
- Remove from the microwave and drain the broccoli.
- In the same pan, melt the remaining coconut oil over medium heat and fry the garlic and ginger for about 1 minute.
- Add the tofu, broccoli and black pepper and cook for 2 minutes, tossing occasionally.
- Remove from the heat and serve hot.

141) Tempeh in tomato sauce

Preparation time: 20 minutes **Cooking time**: 1 hour 20 minutes **Portions**: 4

Ingredients:
- ½ cup of extra virgin olive oil, divided by
- 2 packets of tempeh (8 oz), cut into half-inch horizontal slices
- 1 large yellow onion, chopped
- 3 cloves of garlic, minced
- 1 teaspoon dried oregano, crushed
- 1 teaspoon dried thyme, crushed
- ½ teaspoon of red chilli powder

Directions:
- Preheat the oven to 350 degrees F.
- In a large bowl, add 2 tablespoons of oil and the tempeh slices and stir to coat well.
- In a large frying pan, heat ¼ cup of oil over medium-high heat and cook the tempeh slices for about 5-7 minutes.
- Carefully switch sides and cook for about 5-7 minutes.
- Transfer the cooked tempeh slices to a plate lined with paper towels.
- Set aside to drain.
- Meanwhile, in another non-stick pan, heat the remaining oil over medium-low heat and fry the onion, garlic, herbs and spices for about 8-10 minutes.

Ingredients:
- ½ teaspoon red pepper flakes, crushed
- 1 large green pepper, seeded and thinly sliced
- 1 large yellow pepper, seeded and thinly sliced
- 2 cups fresh tomatoes, finely chopped
- ¼ cup of homemade tomato paste
- 1 teaspoon organic apple cider vinegar
- 1 tablespoon maple syrup
- Add the peppers and fry for about 4-5 minutes, stirring occasionally.
- Add the remaining ingredients and mix until well combined.
- Remove from heat.
- In the bottom of a large casserole dish, arrange the tempeh slices.
- Spread the tomato mixture evenly over the tempeh slices.
- Cover the casserole dish well with a piece of foil.
- Bake for about 1 hour.
- Remove from the oven and set aside to cool slightly.
- Serve hot.

142) South West Stuffed Sweet Potatoes

Preparation time: 30 minutes **Cooking time**: 30 minutes **Portions**: 2

Ingredients:
- 2 sweet potatoes
- 2 tablespoons of coconut oil
- ½ cup of black beans, rinsed and drained
- 1 shallot, sliced
- 3 cups of spinach
- A pinch of dried red pepper
- Pinch of cumin
- 1 avocado, peeled and sliced

Directions:
- Preheat the oven to 400°F/205°C. Clean the sweet potatoes and pierce them several times with a fork. Place the sweet potatoes on a baking sheet lined with baking paper and bake about 50 minutes or until soft.
- Leave the sweet potatoes to cool for 5 minutes.
- While the sweet potatoes are cooling, heat the frying pan over a medium heat and add the coconut oil, shallots and black beans.

Ingredients:
- Condiment
- 3 tablespoons of olive oil
- 1 lime, squeezed
- 1 teaspoon of cumin
- Handful of coriander, chopped
- Salt and pepper

- Cook for 5 minutes then add the spinach, dried chilli flakes and cumin. Cook for another 1 minute.
- In a small bowl, whisk together the dressing ingredients.
- Slice the sweet potatoes in the centre and stuff them with the black bean mixture. Cover with slices of avocado.
- Pour the dressing over the sweet potatoes and serve.

143) Coconut cauliflower with herbs and spices

Preparation time: 30 minutes **Cooking time**: **Portions**: 2

Ingredients:
- ¼ cup of coconut oil, melted
- ½ tablespoon ground cumin
- ¼ teaspoon of ground coriander
- 1 teaspoon ground turmeric
- ¼ teaspoon black pepper, ground
- 1 large cauliflower, cut into small florets

Directions:
- Preheat oven to 425°F/220°C. In a large bowl, mix together coconut oil, cumin, coriander, turmeric and black pepper. Add the cauliflower and stir until well coated.

Ingredients:
- 2 tablespoons of toasted pine nuts
- 1 tablespoon coriander, chopped
- ½ tablespoon mint, coarsely chopped
- 1 tablespoon of sultanas
- Himalayan salt

- Spread the cauliflower on the baking tray and place in the oven for 20 minutes. Remove from the oven and transfer to a serving bowl.
- Mix the pine nuts, coriander, mint, sultanas and salt with the cauliflower and serve hot.

144) Quinoa and Brussels sprouts salad

Preparation time: 5 minutes   **Cooking time**: 0 minutes   **Portions**: 2

Ingredients:
- ¼ cup quinoa, cooked
- ½ pound (227 g) Brussels sprouts, halved, diced, roasted
- 2 tablespoons dried blueberries
- 1 medium white onion, peeled, sliced and caramelised

Directions:
- Take a small bowl, pour in the orange juice and lime juice, add the orange zest and then stir until combined.

Ingredients:
- ⅓ teaspoon of salt
- ⅛ teaspoon of cayenne pepper
- ½ orange, squeezed
- ½ teaspoon of orange peel
- 1 tablespoon lime juice
- Take a salad bowl, put the remaining ingredients in, drizzle with the orange juice mixture and then toss until mixed.
- Serve immediately.

145) Mango and jicama salad

Preparation time: 5 minutes   **Cooking time**: 15 minutes   **Portions**: 1

Ingredients:
- 1 mango, peeled and cut into pieces
- 1 cup of sliced jicama
- 1 cup of sliced pepper

Directions:
- In a small bowl, combine the mango, pepper and jicama.

Ingredients:
- Juice of 1 lime
- 1 tablespoon chilli powder
- Squeeze the lime juice over the vegetables. Sprinkle with chilli powder.
- Refrigerate for 15 minutes to allow the flavours to meld and enjoy.

146) Asparagus and roasted mushroom salad

Preparation time: 10 minutes   **Cooking time**: 15 minutes   **Portions**: 2

Ingredients:
- ½ bunch of asparagus, blunted
- 1 pint of cherry tomatoes
- ½ cup mushrooms, halved
- 1 carrot, peeled and cut into small pieces

Directions:
- Preheat oven to 425ºF (220ºC).
- In a bowl, add the asparagus, tomatoes, mushrooms, carrot and pepper. Add the coconut oil, garlic powder and salt. Stir to coat the vegetables evenly.

Ingredients:
- 1 red or yellow pepper, seeded and cut into small pieces
- 1 tablespoon of coconut oil
- 1 tablespoon garlic powder
- 1 teaspoon sea salt
- Transfer the vegetables to a baking tray, place in the preheated oven and roast for 15 minutes, or until the vegetables are tender.
- Transfer the vegetables to a large bowl. Refrigerate, if desired.
- Divide the vegetables between two bowls and serve hot or cold.

147) Thai green salad

Preparation time: 10 minutes   **Cooking time**: 0 minutes   **Portions**: 2

Ingredients:
- 4 cups chopped iceberg lettuce
- 1 cup of bean sprouts
- 2 carrots, cut into thin slices or spirals
- 1 courgette, cut into thin strips or spirals
- 1 shallot, finely chopped
- 2 tablespoons chopped almonds

Directions:
- In a large bowl, combine the lettuce, bean sprouts, carrots, courgettes, shallots and almonds.

Ingredients:
- Juice of 1 lime
- 1 garlic clove
- 1 teaspoon tamarind paste
- 1 packet of stevia
- ½ teaspoon of sea salt
- In the small bowl of a food processor, add the lime juice, garlic, tamarind, stevia and salt. Blend to combine.
- Pour the dressing over the vegetables and mix well.
- Divide evenly between two bowls and serve.

148) Avocado and quinoa salad

Preparation time: 10 minutes **Cooking time**: 0 minutes **Portions**: 2

Ingredients:
- 1 cup of cooked and cooled quinoa
- 1 avocado, diced
- 1 cup cherry tomatoes, halved
- 1 cup cucumber, peeled and diced
- ¼ cup chopped coriander

Ingredients:
- 1 tablespoon garlic powder
- 1 tablespoon onion powder
- 1 teaspoon sea salt
- 1 tablespoon freshly squeezed lemon juice

Directions:
- In a large bowl, mix together the quinoa, avocado, tomatoes, cucumber, cilantro, garlic powder, onion powder, salt and lemon juice.
- Chill for 15 minutes to allow the flavours to meld.
- Serve immediately or store in the fridge for 2 to 3 days.

149) Caprese salad

Preparation time: 5 minutes **Cooking time**: 0 minutes **Portions**: 2

Ingredients:
- 2 large heirloom tomatoes, sliced
- 1 avocado, sliced

Ingredients:
- 1 bunch of basil leaves
- 1 teaspoon sea salt

Directions:
- n a serving dish, place 1 tomato slice, 1 avocado slice and 1 basil leaf.
- Repeat the pattern with all the remaining tomato slices, avocado slices and basil leaves.
- Salt and serve.

150) Tagliatelle with pumpkin and broccoli salad

Preparation time: 10 minutes **Cooking time:** 50 minutes **Portions:** 4

Ingredients:
- 1 spaghetti squash
- 2 tablespoons of coconut oil
- 2 cups of cooked broccoli florets
- 1 red pepper, seedless and cut into strips
- 1 shallot, chopped

Ingredients:
- 1 tablespoon sesame oil
- 1 teaspoon of red pepper flakes
- 2 teaspoons of sea salt, divided
- 2 tablespoons of toasted sesame seeds

Directions:
- Preheat the oven to 350°F (180°C).
- To roast a pumpkin, cut it in half lengthways and scrape out the seeds. Brush each half with coconut oil and season with 1 teaspoon of sea salt. Place the pumpkin halves with the cut side up on a baking tray and roast in the preheated oven for about 50 minutes, or until tender to the fork.
- Prepare the pumpkin noodles by removing the inside of the roasted pumpkin with a fork in a large bowl.
- Add the broccoli, red pepper and shallot.
- In a small bowl, combine the sesame oil, red pepper flakes and remaining salt. Pour over the vegetables. Stir gently to combine.
- Garnish with sesame seeds and serve.

151) Broccoli and mandarin salad

Preparation time: 5 minutes **Cooking time**: 0 minutes **Portions**: 4

Ingredients:
- 4 cups of cooked and cooled broccoli florets
- 2 mandarins without seeds, peeled and separated
- ⅓ cup of freshly squeezed orange juice
- 2 tablespoons of sesame oil

Ingredients:
- 2 cloves of garlic, minced
- ½ teaspoon of sea salt
- ¼ teaspoon red pepper flakes

Directions:
- In a large bowl, combine the broccoli and tangerine sections.
- In a blender, combine the orange juice, sesame oil, garlic, salt and red pepper flakes. Blend until smooth.
- Pour the dressing over the broccoli salad. Refrigerate for 1 hour to blend the flavours.
- Serve cold.

152) Spinach and mushroom salad

Preparation time: 2 minutes   **Cooking time**: 5 minutes   **Portions**: 2

Ingredients:
- 1 (6-ounce / 170-g) packet of baby spinach leaves
- ½ cup of roasted and ground almonds
- 1 tablespoon sesame oil
- 1 tablespoon apple cider vinegar

Directions:
- In a large bowl, combine the spinach and almonds.
- In a small saucepan over low heat, combine the sesame oil, cider vinegar, salt and mushrooms.

Ingredients:
- 1 teaspoon sea salt
- 1 cup chopped shiitake mushrooms
- Water, as required

- Cook for about 5 minutes, or until the mushrooms are softened, adding water if necessary.
- Pour the mushroom dressing over the spinach. Stir well to coat the spinach leaves.
- Serve immediately.

153) Broccoli, asparagus and quinoa salad

Preparation time: 5 minutes   **Cooking time**: 0 minutes   **Portions**: 4

Ingredients:
- 1 cup of cooked broccoli florets, coarsely chopped
- 1 cup asparagus, cut and cooked, coarsely chopped
- 2 cups of cooked and cooled quinoa
- ½ cup of water

Directions:
- In a large bowl, combine the broccoli and asparagus.
- Stir in the quinoa.
- In a blender, combine the water, lemon juice, coconut oil and salt.
- Blend until the ingredients are emulsified.

Ingredients:
- 2 tablespoons freshly squeezed lemon juice
- 2 tablespoons of coconut oil
- ½ teaspoon of sea salt

- Pour the dressing over the salad. Stir to combine.
- Refrigerate the salad for 15 minutes to chill.
- Serve cold.

154) Root salad

Preparation time: 15 minutes   **Cooking time**: 0 minutes   **Portions**: 2

Ingredients:
- 1 red beet, peeled and chopped
- 1 golden beetroot, peeled and chopped
- 2 carrots, peeled and cut into pieces

Directions:
- In a medium bowl, mix together the red beetroot, golden beetroot, carrots, hazelnuts, sultanas and salt.

Ingredients:
- 2 tablespoons hazelnuts
- 2 tablespoons of sultanas
- ½ teaspoon of sea salt

- Refrigerate for 15 minutes to blend the flavours. Serve.

155) Lush summer salad

Preparation time: 5 minutes   **Cooking time**: 0 minutes   **Portions**: 4

Ingredients:
- 4 cups chopped iceberg or romaine lettuce
- 2 cups cherry tomatoes, halved
- 1 (14.5-ounce / 411-g) can of whole green beans, drained
- ½ cup of shredded carrot

Directions:
- In a large bowl, combine the lettuce, tomatoes, green beans, carrot, shallot, cucumber and radishes.

Ingredients:
- 1 shallot, sliced
- 1 cucumber, peeled and sliced
- 2 radishes, thinly sliced

- Mix well with 2 tablespoons of the seasoning of your choice and serve immediately.

156) Salad of sea vegetables and algae

Preparation time: 5 minutes   **Cooking time**: 0 minutes   **Portions**: 2

Ingredients:
- ✓ 1 cup of dried sea vegetables
- ✓ 1 ounce (28 g) of dried seaweed
- ✓ 1 teaspoon spirulina

Directions:
- ❖ Reconstitute the sea vegetables and dried seaweed according to the package directions.
- ❖ Meanwhile, in a small bowl, mix together the spirulina, cider vinegar and stevia.

Ingredients:
- ✓ 1 teaspoon apple cider vinegar
- ✓ 1 packet of stevia
- ✓ 1 teaspoon of sesame seeds

- ❖ Drain the sea vegetables and seaweed. Squeeze out excess moisture and place in a medium bowl. Add the spirulina mixture and mix.
- ❖ Refrigerate for 1 hour to blend the flavours.
- ❖ Add sesame seeds and serve.

157) Rainbow salad

Preparation time: 10 minutes   **Cooking time:** 0 minutes   **Portions:** 2

Ingredients:
- ✓ 1 mango, peeled, boned and diced
- ✓ ¼ onion, chopped
- ✓ ½ cup cherry tomatoes, halved
- ✓ ½ cucumber, seedless, sliced

Directions:
- ❖ Take a medium bowl, place the mango pieces in it, add the onion, tomatoes, cucumber and pepper and then drizzle with lime juice.

Ingredients:
- ✓ ½ of a green pepper, seedless, sliced
- ✓ ⅓ teaspoon of salt
- ✓ ¼ teaspoon cayenne pepper
- ✓ ¼ key lime, squeezed

- ❖ Season with salt and cayenne pepper, mix until combined, and leave the salad in the fridge for a minimum of 20 minutes.
- ❖ Serve immediately.

158) Rocket salad with basil

Preparation time: 5 minutes   **Cooking time:** 10 minutes   **Portions:** 2

Ingredients:
- ✓ 4 ounces (113 g) arugula
- ✓ ½ cup cherry tomatoes, halved
- ✓ ¼ cup of basil leaves
- ✓ ½ key lime, squeezed

Directions:
- ❖ Prepare the dressing and for this, take a small bowl, put the lime juice in it, add the tahini butter, salt and cayenne pepper and then whisk until combined.

Ingredients:
- ✓ 2 tablespoons of walnuts
- ✓ ¼ teaspoon of salt
- ✓ ⅛ teaspoon of cayenne pepper
- ✓ ½ tablespoon of tahini butter

- ❖ Take a medium bowl, put the rocket, tomatoes and basil leaves in it, pour in the dressing and then massage with your hands.
- ❖ Let the salad stand for 20 minutes, then taste to adjust the dressing and serve.

159) Green cucumber and rocket salad

Preparation time: 5 minutes   **Cooking time:** 0 minutes   **Portions:** 2

Ingredients:
- ✓ ½ cucumber, seedless
- ✓ 4 ounces (113 g) arugula
- ✓ ⅛ teaspoon of salt

Directions:
- ❖ Slice the cucumber, add it to a salad bowl and then add the rocket.

Ingredients:
- ✓ 1 tablespoon lime juice
- ✓ 1 tablespoon olive oil
- ✓ ⅛ teaspoon of cayenne pepper

- ❖ Mix together the lime juice and oil until combined, pour over the salad and then season with salt and cayenne pepper.
- ❖ Stir until combined and then serve.

160) Strawberry and dandelion salad

Preparation time: 10 minutes **Cooking time**: 7 minutes **Portions**: 2

Ingredients:
- ½ onion, peeled, sliced
- 5 strawberries, sliced
- 2 cups dandelion tops, rinsed

Ingredients:
- 1 tablespoon lime juice
- 1 tablespoon of grape oil
- ¼ teaspoon of salt

Directions:
- Take a medium frying pan, place it over medium heat, add the oil and let it heat until hot.
- Add the onion, season with ⅛ teaspoon salt, stir until combined, and then cook for 3 to 5 minutes until tender and golden.
- In the meantime, take a small bowl, place the strawberry slices in it, drizzle with ½ tablespoon of lime juice and then toss until coated.
- When the onions have turned golden, add the remaining lime juice, stir until combined, and then cook for 1 minute.
- Remove the pan from the heat, transfer the onions to a large salad bowl, add the strawberries with their juice and the dandelion, and then sprinkle with the remaining salt. Stir until combined and then serve.

161) Wakame and pepper salad

Preparation time: 15 minutes **Cooking time**: 0 minutes **Portions**: 2

Ingredients:
- 1 cup of wakame stalks
- ½ tablespoon chopped red pepper
- ½ teaspoon of onion powder
- ½ tablespoon lime juice

Ingredients:
- ½ tablespoon agave syrup
- ½ tablespoon sesame seeds
- ½ tablespoon sesame oil

Directions:
- Put the wakame stalks in a bowl, cover with water, let them soak for 10 minutes and then drain.
- Meanwhile, prepare the dressing and for this, take a small bowl, add the lime juice, onion, agave syrup and sesame oil and then whisk until combined.
- Place the drained wakame stalks in a large dish, add the pepper, pour in the seasoning and stir until coated.
- Sprinkle the salad with sesame seeds and serve.

DINNER

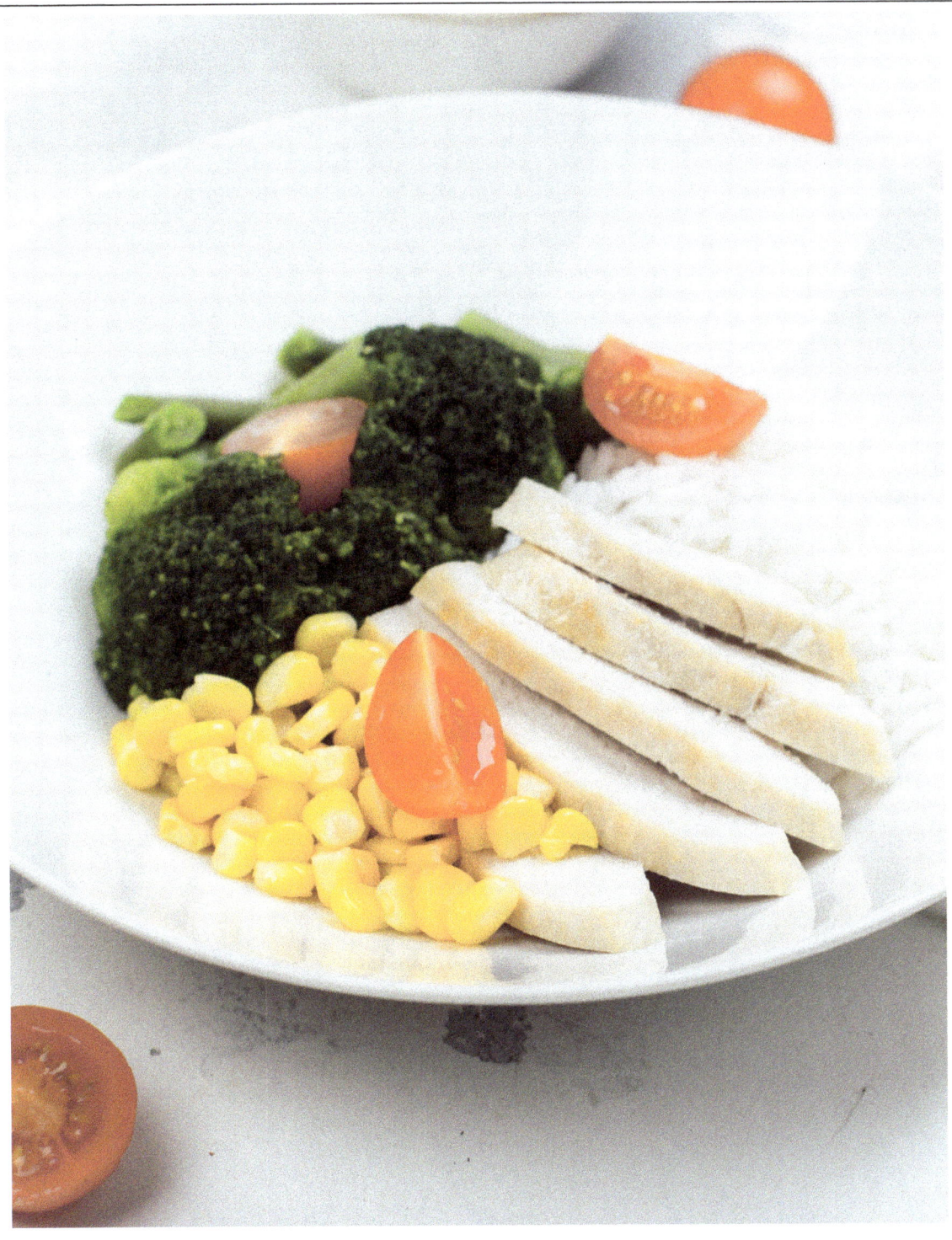

162) Carrot and potato stew with herbs

Preparation time: 10 minutes   **Cooking time**: 50 minutes   **Portions**: 4 people

Ingredients:
- ✓ 1 tablespoon avocado oil
- ✓ 1 cup onion, diced
- ✓ 2 cloves of garlic, crushed
- ✓ 1 teaspoon sea salt
- ✓ 1 teaspoon freshly ground black pepper
- ✓ 3 cups vegetable stock, more if desired

Ingredients:
- ✓ 2 cups of water, plus more if desired
- ✓ 3 cups of sliced carrots
- ✓ 1 large potato, diced
- ✓ 2 stalks of celery, diced
- ✓ 1 teaspoon dried oregano
- ✓ 1 dried bay leaf

Directions:
- ❖ In a medium saucepan over medium heat, heat the avocado oil. Add the onion, garlic, salt and pepper, and sauté for 2 to 3 minutes, or until the onion is soft.
- ❖ Add the vegetable stock, water, carrot, potato, celery, oregano and bay leaf and stir. Bring to the boil, reduce the heat to medium-low and cook for 30-45 minutes, or until the potatoes and carrots are tender.
- ❖ Adjust the seasonings, if necessary, and add more water or vegetable stock if you prefer a softer consistency, in half-cup increments.
- ❖ Pour into 4 soup bowls and enjoy.

163) Berry and mint soup

Preparation time: 5 minutes   **Cooking time**: 0 minutes   **Portions**: 1 to 2

Ingredients:
- ✓ ¼ cup of unrefined whole cane sugar, such as Sucanat
- ✓ ¼ cup of water, more if desired
- ✓ 1 cup mixed berries (raspberries, blackberries, blueberries)

Ingredients:
- ✓ ½ cup of water
- ✓ 1 teaspoon freshly squeezed lemon juice
- ✓ 8 fresh mint leaves

Directions:
- ❖ In a small saucepan over medium-low heat, heat the sugar and water, stirring constantly for 1 to 2 minutes, until the sugar is dissolved. Cool.
- ❖ In a blender, blend together the cooled sugar water with the berries, water, lemon juice and mint leaves until well combined.
- ❖ Transfer the mixture to the refrigerator and allow it to cool completely, about 20 minutes.
- ❖ Pour into 1 large or 2 small bowls and enjoy.

164) Potato and broccoli soup

Preparation time: 10 minutes **Cooking time:** 25 minutes **Servings: 2 to 1**

Ingredients:
- 1 tablespoon avocado oil
- ½ cup diced onion
- 2 cloves of garlic, crushed
- 3 cups vegetable stock
- 1 (13.5-ounce / 383-g) can of whole coconut milk

Directions:
- In a large frying pan over medium-high heat, heat the avocado oil. Add the onion and garlic and fry for 2 to 3 minutes, or until the onions are soft.
- Add the vegetable stock, coconut milk, potatoes, broccoli, salt and pepper and continue to cook for 18-20 minutes, or until the potatoes are soft. Remove from the heat and cool.

Ingredients:
- 2 cups potatoes, peeled and diced
- 3 cups of chopped broccoli florets
- 1 teaspoon sea salt
- 1½ teaspoons of freshly ground black pepper

- In a blender, blend the cooled soup until smooth.
- Adjust seasonings as necessary. Pour into 2 large or 4 small bowls and enjoy.

165) Lush pepper soup

Preparation time: 5 minutes **Cooking time:** 10 minutes **Servings: 2 to 4**

Ingredients:
- 1 teaspoon avocado oil
- ¼ cup diced onions
- 2 cloves of garlic, crushed
- 2 cups of diced red peppers
- 2 cups of vegetable stock

Directions:
- In a frying pan over medium-high heat, add the avocado oil, onions, garlic and red peppers and fry for 2 to 3 minutes, or until the onions are soft; allow to cool.
- In a blender, blend together the sauté, vegetable stock, jalapeño and salt until well combined and completely liquid; adjust the seasonings according to your preference.

Ingredients:
- ½ to 1 jalapeño, seeded and diced
- 1 teaspoon sea salt
- ½ cup diced red peppers
- ½ cup of diced yellow peppers

- Transfer the soup to a medium bowl and toss it with the diced red and yellow peppers.
- Cover and refrigerate for 20-30 minutes to cool or chill overnight.
- Pour into 2 large or 4 small bowls and enjoy.

166) Cabbage and yellow onion soup

Preparation time: 10 minutes **Cooking time:** 20 minutes **Servings: 2 to 4**

Ingredients:
- 1 tablespoon avocado oil
- 2 cups thinly sliced yellow onions (3 medium)
- 1 teaspoon unrefined whole cane sugar, such as Sucanat
- 1 cup of vegetable stock
- 2 cups of water

Directions:
- In a medium saucepan over medium-high heat, heat the avocado oil. Add the onions and sauté for 3-5 minutes, or until the onions start to get soft.
- Add the sugar and continue to fry, stirring constantly, for 8-10 minutes, or until the onions are slightly caramelised.

Ingredients:
- 2 tablespoons of coconut amino acids
- 2 cloves of garlic, crushed
- ½ teaspoon dried thyme
- ½ teaspoon of sea salt
- 3 cabbage stalks, shredded and cut into ribbons (approx. 2 cups)

- Add the vegetable stock, water, coconut amino acid, garlic, thyme and salt. Reduce the heat to medium-low and simmer for 5-7 minutes. Adjust seasonings as necessary.
- Add the cabbage and leave on the heat just long enough for it to wilt.
- Remove from the heat, pour into 2 large or 4 small bowls and serve.

167) Wild rice, mushroom and leek soup

Preparation time: 10 minutes **Cooking time:** 55 minutes **Portions: 1 to 2**

Ingredients:
- ⅓ cup of wild rice
- 1 cup of sliced cremini mushrooms
- ½ cup of sliced leeks, only the white part
- 3 cups of water

Directions:
- Prepare the wild rice according to the package instructions.
- In a medium saucepan over high heat, bring the sliced mushrooms, leeks and water to the boil. Boil for 8-10 minutes, or until the mushrooms are soft.

Ingredients:
- 2 tablespoons of organic white miso
- ¼ to ½ teaspoon of freshly ground black pepper
- Sliced shallots, for garnish

- Add the cooked wild rice, miso and black pepper. Using the back side of a spoon, mash the miso on the side of the pot to break it up, then stir it in.
- Remove from the heat. Pour into 1 large or 2 small bowls, garnish with chopped shallots and enjoy.

168) Pear and ginger soup

Preparation time: 10 minutes **Cooking time:** 15 minutes **Portions: 1 to 2**

Ingredients:
- 2 teaspoons of avocado oil
- ½ cup diced onions
- 2 cloves of garlic, crushed
- 1 cup of vegetable stock
- 2 cups of water
- ¼ cup of coconut milk (canned)

Directions:
- In a large frying pan over medium-high heat, heat the avocado oil. Add the onion and garlic and fry for 2 to 3 minutes, or until the onions are soft.
- Add the vegetable stock, water, coconut milk, pears, ginger and salt and cook over a medium-high heat for 8-10 minutes, or until the pears are soft. Remove from the heat and cool.

Ingredients:
- 2 pears, peeled and diced
- 1 inch fresh ginger root, chopped
- ¼ teaspoon of sea salt
- Sliced radishes, for garnish (optional)
- Chopped shallots, for garnish (optional)

- Transfer the soup to a blender and blend until well combined. Adjust seasonings as necessary.
- Pour immediately into 1 large or 2 small bowls, garnish with the radishes and shallots (if using), and enjoy, or return the soup to the stove to warm slightly over low heat before serving.

169) Asparagus and artichoke soup

Preparation time: 5 minutes **Cooking time:** 20 minutes **Servings: 4 cups**

Ingredients:
- ½ cup diced onion
- 1 tablespoon avocado oil
- 2 cloves of garlic, crushed
- 1 cup of diced potatoes
- 8 asparagus stalks, cut into small pieces

Directions:
- In a medium frying pan, fry the onion, avocado oil and garlic over medium-high heat for 2 to 3 minutes, or until the onion is soft.
- Transfer the sauté to a medium-sized saucepan and add the potatoes, asparagus, vegetable stock, salt and pepper; cook over medium-high heat for 18 to 20 minutes, or until the potatoes are tender. Add more vegetable stock, if necessary, to keep the liquid level between ½ and 1 inch above the contents of the saucepan. Remove from heat and let cool.

Ingredients:
- 2 cups of vegetable stock
- ½ to ¾ teaspoon of sea salt
- ½ teaspoon ground black pepper
- 2 cups of almond milk
- 1 tin of artichoke hearts, cut in half and with stem

- In a blender, blend the cooled soup mixture, the almond milk and the artichokes until everything is well combined and the soup is smooth. Adjust the seasonings to your liking and add more almond milk or vegetable stock to thin it out, if you prefer.
- Return the soup to the saucepan and heat slightly over low heat before serving.

170) Carrot and celery soup

Preparation time: 15 minutes **Cooking time:** 1 hour and 10 minutes **Portions: 4 people**

Ingredients:
- Cooking spray
- 1 large onion, coarsely chopped
- 2 large carrots, peeled and roughly chopped
- 2 large celery stalks (with leaves), roughly chopped
- 1 parsnip, peeled and roughly chopped

Directions:
- Spray the bottom of a large saucepan with cooking spray. Put the pan over medium-low heat, add the onion and sauté for about 5 minutes, stirring constantly.
- Add the carrots, celery, parsnips, garlic and leek to the pot. Fry for a further 3 minutes.

Ingredients:
- 5 cloves of garlic, crushed
- 1 leek, well cleaned and coarsely chopped
- 9 cups of water
- 2 bay leaves
- 2 teaspoons of sea salt

- Add the water, bay leaf and salt. Simmer for 1 hour.
- Remove from the heat and cool slightly. Drain the vegetables, leaving only the stock.
- To serve, add back some of the vegetables if you like and heat the soup to the desired temperature.

171) Creamy clam chowder with mushrooms

Preparation time: 15 minutes **Cooking time:** 30 minutes **Portions: 4**

Ingredients:
- For the clams with mushrooms:
- ½ cup coarsely chopped shiitake mushrooms
- 1 teaspoon of coconut oil
- ¼ cup of water
- ½ teaspoon celery seeds
- For the soup base:
- ½ medium onion, chopped
- 3 medium-sized carrots, peeled and chopped
- 2 stalks of celery, finely chopped

Directions:
- To make clams with mushrooms
- In a large saucepan over medium-high heat, add the mushrooms and coconut oil. Sauté for 3 minutes. Add the water and celery seeds, stirring until the water is absorbed.
- Remove from the heat and transfer the mushrooms to a plate.
- To make the soup base
- In the same pot, over a medium heat, sauté the onion, carrots, celery and thyme for about 5 minutes, or until the onion is softened. Add a little stock if necessary.

Ingredients:
- 1 teaspoon dried thyme
- 3 cups vegetable stock
- 1 sheet of nori, finely crumbled
- For the cream base:
- 1 cup lightly steamed cauliflower
- ¾ cup of unsweetened almond milk
- ¼ teaspoon of sea salt

- Then, add the remaining stock and nori and bring to the boil.
- To make the cream base
- In a blender or food processor, add the cauliflower, almond milk and salt. Blend to combine. If the mixture is too thick, add a little soup base to thin it out. Blend until the mixture is smooth.
- To assemble the fish soup
- Add the mushroom mix and the cream base to the soup base. Stir well to combine.
- Heat for 5 minutes, or until hot, and serve.

172) Bok choy soup, broccolini and brown rice

Preparation time: 5 minutes **Cooking time:** 10 minutes **Portions: 2**

Ingredients:
- 3 cups vegetable stock
- 1 cup of chopped bok choy

Ingredients:
- 1 bunch of broccolini, roughly chopped
- ½ cup cooked brown rice

Directions:
- In a medium saucepan over medium heat, place the stock, bok choy, broccolini and brown rice. Bring to the boil and cook for 10 minutes, or until the vegetables are cooked through and tender. Serve.

173) Apple and sweet pumpkin soup

Preparation time: 5 minutes **Cooking time**: 25 minutes **Serves 2**

Ingredients:
- ✓ 1 medium apple, core and slices
- ✓ ½ cup chopped fennel
- ✓ 1½ cups of water, divided
- ✓ 1 cup unsweetened canned pumpkin puree
- ✓ ¾ cup low-sodium vegetable broth
- ✓ 4 small, pitted dates
- ✓ 2 teaspoons of freshly grated ginger or 2 cubes of frozen ginger

Ingredients:
- ✓ ¼ teaspoon ground cinnamon
- ✓ ¼ teaspoon of curry powder
- ✓ ⅛ teaspoon dried thyme
- ✓ ⅛ teaspoon of sea salt
- ✓ ⅛ teaspoon of ground cumin
- ✓ 4 teaspoons of sultanas, for garnish
- ✓ 2 teaspoons of fennel seeds, toasted, for garnish

Directions:
- ❖ In a saucepan, combine the apples, fennel and ½ cup water. Cover and simmer for about 25 minutes, until the apples and fennel are softened.
- ❖ In a food processor, combine the apple and fennel mixture, pumpkin, remaining 1 cup water, stock, dates, ginger, cinnamon, curry powder, thyme, salt and cumin. Process until reduced to a puree.
- ❖ Pour the soup into two bowls and cover each with 2 teaspoons of sultanas and 1 teaspoon of toasted fennel seeds.
- ❖ Serve immediately or allow to cool and serve at room temperature.

174) Tomato and carrot soup with lemon

Preparation time: 5 minutes **Cooking time**: 35 minutes **Portions: 2**

Ingredients:
- ✓ 1 (15-ounce / 425-g) may no sodium added diced tomatoes, drained
- ✓ ¾ cup chopped carrots
- ✓ 1 tablespoon avocado oil
- ✓ ¼ teaspoon of sea salt

Ingredients:
- ✓ 1 cup of water
- ✓ ½ cup low-sodium vegetable broth
- ✓ 2 tablespoons fresh coriander, chopped
- ✓ 1 tablespoon freshly squeezed lemon juice

Directions:
- ❖ Preheat the oven to 400°F (205°C).
- ❖ In a glass baking dish, combine the tomatoes, carrots, oil and salt and mix well.
- ❖ Cook the tomato and carrot mixture for 35 minutes, or until caramelised, then carefully transfer to a food processor.
- ❖ Add the water and stock and whisk until smooth.
- ❖ Garnish with coriander and add lemon juice to taste.

175) Courgette and avocado soup with basil

Preparation time: 5 minutes **Cooking time**: 0 minutes **Serves 2**

Ingredients:
- ✓ 2 large courgettes, chopped
- ✓ 1 medium avocado
- ✓ 1 medium pepper
- ✓ ½ cup low-sodium vegetable broth
- ✓ ½ cup of water
- ✓ ¼ cup chopped fennel

Ingredients:
- ✓ 6 fresh basil leaves, plus 2 small leaves for garnish
- ✓ 2 teaspoons fresh rosemary, chopped
- ✓ 1 clove of garlic, peeled, or 1 frozen garlic cube
- ✓ ⅛ teaspoon of sea salt
- ✓ 1½ teaspoons of hulled pumpkin seeds, toasted, for garnish

Directions:
- ❖ In a high-speed blender or food processor, combine the courgettes, avocado, pepper, stock, water, fennel, basil, rosemary, garlic and salt and blend until pureed.
- ❖ Pour the soup into bowls. Garnish each with a small basil leaf and pumpkin seeds and serve.

176) Courgette, spinach and quinoa soup

Preparation time: 5 minutes **Cooking time:** 25 minutes **Portions: 4 people**

Ingredients:
- ✓ 2 tablespoons of avocado oil
- ✓ ¼ teaspoon dried oregano
- ✓ ¼ teaspoon dried thyme
- ✓ ⅛ teaspoon of sea salt
- ✓ 1 large onion, chopped
- ✓ 2 large courgettes, peeled and cut into pieces

Directions:
- ❖ In a soup pot, heat the oil over medium heat for 1 minute, then add the oregano, thyme and salt and cook for 30 seconds.
- ❖ Add the onion, cover and cook for 7-8 minutes, stirring regularly, until softened.
- ❖ Add the courgettes. Cook for a further 12 minutes, or until the courgettes are soft.

Ingredients:
- ✓ 1 cup of low-sodium vegetable broth
- ✓ 1 cup of water
- ✓ 1 cup baby spinach
- ✓ 6 large fresh basil leaves
- ✓ ⅓ cup of cooked quinoa (optional)
- ✓ Juice of 1 lemon
- ❖ Add the stock and water and cook for a further 3 minutes, until heated through.
- ❖ Add the spinach and basil and cook until just wilted.
- ❖ Transfer the mixture to a food processor and process until it is pureed.
- ❖ Add quinoa (if using). Season with lemon juice and serve.

177) Easy Cilantro Lime Quinoa.

Preparation time: 5 minutes **Cooking time:** 15 minutes **Portions: 6**

Ingredients:
- ✓ 1 cup quinoa, rinsed and draned.
- ✓ ½ cup fresh cilantro, chopped
- ✓ 1 lime zest, grated

Directions:
- ❖ Add quinoa and water to the instant pot and stir well.
- ❖ Seal with a lid and select manual mode and set the timer for 5 minutes.

Ingredients:
- ✓ 2 tbsp. fresh lime juice
- ✓ 1 ¼ cup distilled water feed Sea sa sa

- ❖ Once finished, allow pressure naturally release that open thed.
- ❖ Stir in water, leave to rest.
- ❖ Season with salt and serve.

178) Spinach Quinoa

Preparation time: 10 minutes **Cooking time:** 25 minutes **Portions: 4**

Ingredients:
- ✓ 1 cup quinoa
- ✓ 2 cups fresh spinach, chopped
- ✓ 1 ½ cups filtered alkaline water
- ✓ 1 sweet potato, peeled and cut into pieces
- ✓ 1 tsp. coriander powder
- ✓ 1 teaspoon turmandine
- ✓ 1 teaspoon of cumin seds

Directions:
- ❖ Add oil il instant pot and set the sauté mode.
- ❖ Add onion in olive oil and fry for 2 minutes otil onion is softened.
- ❖ Add garlic, ginger, spices and quinoa and coook for 3-4 minutes.
- ❖ Add spinach, sweet potatoes, and water and stir well.

Ingredients:
- ✓ 1 tsp. fresh ginger, chopped
- ✓ 2 garlic cloves, chopped
- ✓ 1 onion cut in half
- ✓ 2 tbsp olive oil
- ✓ 1 fresh lime juice
- ✓ Pepper Salt

- ❖ Cook at high pressure for 2 minutes.
- ❖ When it's finished, release the pressure naturally and then open the container. Add the lime juice and mix well.
- ❖ Serve and enjoy.

179) Healthy broccoli Asparagus Soup

Preparation time: 15 minutes. **Cooking time**: 28 minutes. **Portions: 6**

Ingredients:
- 2 cups broccoli florets, chopped
- 15 asparages spears, escreated and chopped
- 1 tsp. dried oregano
- 1 tbsp. fresh thyme leaves
- ½ cup unsweetened almond milk

Directions:
- Add the oil to the bowl and stir the bowl.
- Add onion to olive oil and fry until onion is softened.
- Add the garlic and leave to stand for 30 minutes.
- Add all the vegetables and salt and dry well.

Ingredients:
- 3 ½ cups filtered alkaline water
- 2 cups cauliflower florets, chopped
- 2 tsp. garlic, chopped 1 cup onion, chopped
- 2 tbsp. olive oil
- Salt Pepper
- Seal pot with lid and coook on manual mode for 3 minutes.
- Once finished, you can rinse to minimise pressure and then close the container.
- Puree the soup with an immersion blender until smooth. Add the almond milk, herbs, pepper and salt.
- Serve and enjoy.

180) Creamy Asparagus Soup

Preparation time: 10 minutes **Cooking time**: 40 minutes **Portions: 6**

Ingredients:
- 2 lbs. fresh asparagus cut off woody stems
- ¼ tablespoon lemon zest
- 2 tbsp. lime juice
- 14 oz. coconut milk
- 1 tsp. tied thyme.
- ½ tsp. oregano
- ½ tsp. sage

Directions:
- Preheat the oven to 400°F/ 200°C.
- The paper tray with the scraps and leftovers.
- Arrange the asparagus spears on a baking tray. Add 2 tbsp of walnut oil and add salt, seasonings, garlic and sugar.
- Kiss it with a dose of 20-25 mnutes.
- Add the remaining oil in the instant pot and set the pot on sauté mode.
- Add the garlic and milk to the pot and fry for 2-3 minutes.

Ingredients:
- 1 ½ cups alkaline water filtered.
- 1 Head of a hunting dog coming out of the floor.
- 1 tablespoon. garlic, minced
- 1 leek, sliced
- 3 tbsp. coconut oil
- Pinch of Himalayan salt.
- Add the cauliflower florets and water to the bowl and mix well.
- Insert the cooker with a rod and select steam and let it stand for 4 minutes.
- When finished, release the pressure using the quick-release method.
- Add roasted asparagus, lime zest, lime juice, and coco milk and stir well.
- Puree the soup with an immersion blender until it is pureed.
- Serve and have fun

181) Spicy Eggplant

Preparation time: 15 minutes **Cooking time**: 5 minutes **Portions: 4**

Ingredients:
- 1 aubergine, cut into 1inch cubes
- ½ cup filtered alkaline water
- 1 life, in book form.
- ½ tsp. Italian seasoning
- 1 tsp. paprika

Directions:
- Add the extract and salt to the instant flour.
- Cook on manual high pressure for 5 minutes.
- When finished, rinse with peanut butter and then milk. Wet the aubergines well.

Ingredients:
- ½ tsp. red pepper
- 1 tsp. garlic powder
- 2 tbsp. olive oil extra virgin
- ¼ teaspoon of sea salt
- Add oil to the Instant Pot and set pot on sauté mode.
- Put the ingredient back into the pot with the chopper, garlic, paprika and salt and mix until it is included.
- Coook on sauté mode for 5 minutes. Stir from time to time.
- Serve enjoy.

182) Brussels Sprouts and carrots

Preparation time: 10 minutes **Cooking time**: 5 minutes **Portions**: 6

Ingredients:
- 1 ½ pounds of Brussels sprouts, trimmed and cut alf
- 4 carrots peel and cut slices are shaped like a knife.
- 1 tsp. olive oil
- ½ cup filtered alkaline water
- 1 tbsp. dried parsley

Directions:
- Add all ingredients to the instant pot and mix well.
- Put the lid on the pan and cook over a high heat for 2 minutes.

Ingredients:
- ¼ tsp. garlic, minced
- ¼ tsp. pepper
- ¼ tsp. sea salt

- When finished, rinse with the quick-release button and then with the lid.
- Stir well all serve.

183) Matured Cajun Zucchini

Preparation time: 8 minutes. **Cooking time**: 2 minutes. **Portions**: 2

Ingredients:
- 4 zucchinis, sliced
- 1 tsp. garlic powder
- 1 tsp. paprika

Directions:
- Add all the ingredients to the pot and mix well.
- Close the cooker with the lid and cook at low pressure for 1 minute.

Ingredients:
- 2 tbsp. Cajun seasoning
- ½ cup melted milk water
- 1 tablespoon olive oil

- Once finished, release the pressure using the quick-release method then opene the lid.
- Mix well and serve.

- 130 Fat: 7.9 Carbohydrates: 14.7 g. Sugar: 7.2 g. Protein: 5.3 g. Cholesterol: 0 mg.

184) Fried cabage

Preparation time: 10 minutes **Cooking time**: 3 minutes **Portions**: 6

Ingredients:
- 1 head cabbage, chopped
- ½ teaspoon of olive oil
- ½ onion, diced
- ½ tsp. paprika

Directions:
- Add olive oil il inside the Instant Pot and set the sauté mode.
- Add onion in olive oil and sauté until soft.
- Add the ingredients for preparation and the product for packaging.

Ingredients:
- 1 onion, chopped
- 1 fibreglass basket
- 2 tbsp. olive oil
- ½ tbsp sea salt

- Close the lid and cook over a high heat for 3 minutes.
- When you're finished, release the pressure using the quick-release method then open the lids.
- Mix well and serve.

185) Tofu Curry

Preparation time: 10 minutes **Cooking time**: 4 hours **Portions**: 4

Ingredients:
- 1 cup firm tofu, diced
- 2 tbsp garlic cloves, minced
- 1 onion, chopped
- 8 oz. tomato pured
- 2 cups pepper, chopped

Directions:
- Add all ingredients except tofu in a blender and blend until smooth.
- Put the blended mixture into the Instant Pot.

Ingredients:
- 1 tablespoon garm masala
- 2 tbsp. olive oil
- 1 tablespoon peanut butter
- 10 oz. coconut milk
- 1 ½ tsp. sea salt

- Add the tofu to a bowl and dry it well.
- Seal pot with a lid and select slow coook mode and set the timer for 4 hours.
- Mix well and serve.

186) Cauliflower with sauce

Preparation time: 10 minutes **Cooking time:** 15 minutes **Portions:** 5

Ingredients:
- 1 large bed cauliflower head, cut bottom leaves
  For marinade:
- 1 tsp. paprika ½ tbsp olive oil
- Tbsp. fresh parsley, chopped
- 1 tbsp. thyme fresh
- 3 garlic cloves
- Salt Pepper

Directions:
- In a full bowl, mix all the marinade ingredints.
- Rub the marinade evenly over the entire head of the cauliflower.
- For gravy: add oil instant pot and set the pot on sauté modeuté.
- Add the garlic and onion in oil olive oil and sauté until the onion is softened.
- Add the water, lemon juice and thyme and stir.
- Place the trivet in the Instant Pot. Place the cauliflower in the trivet.

Ingredients:
- For gravy:
- ½ tbsp. lime juice
- ½ teaspoon
- 1 ½ cups filtered alkaline water
- 2 cloves garlic
- 1 tsp. olive oil
- 1 onion, diced
- Seal the pot with lid and coook on manual high pressure for 3 minutes.
- When finished, allow to release naturally pressure for 5 minutes then release using a quick-release method. Transfer the cauliflower head to a serving dish and salt for 3-4 minutes.
- Reduce the Instant Pot to a puree with an immersion blender until it reaches consistency.
- Put some of the herb on a frying pan and cook the meat for 3-4 minutes.
- Serve the cauliflower with gravy.

187) Zucchini Noodles

Preparation time: 8 minutes **Cooking time:** 2 minutes **Portions:** 2

Ingredients:
- 2 large courgettes, spiralised
- 1 tbsp. fresh mint leaves, sliced
- 1/3 lime juice
- ½ lime zest

Directions:
- Add oil instant pot and seet the pot outé.
- Add the lime zest, garlic and salt to the olive oil and leave to dry for 30 minutes.

Ingredients:
- 2 garlic cloves, chopped
- 2 tbsp. olive oil
- ¼ tsp. pepper
- ½ tsp. sea salt
- Add the zucchini noodles and lime juice and stir for 30 seconds. Season with pepper and salt. Season with milk.
- Serve and enjoy.

188) Buckwheat Porridge

Preparation time: 20 minutes **Cooking time:** 10 minutes **Portions:** 4

Ingredients:
- 1 cup buckwheat groats, rinsed
- 2 tablespoons almonds, chopped
- ½ tsp. vanilla

Directions:
- Add the peanut butter, vanilla, cinnamon and milk to the instant water and mix well.
- Close the cooker with the lid and cook at manual high pressure for 6 minutes.

Ingredients:
- 1 tsp. cinnamon
- 3 cups untreated almond milk
- 4-5 drops liquid stevia.
- Once finished, let release pressure naturally then open the lid.
- Top with chopped almonds and serve.

189) Vegetable soup

Preparation time: 15 minutes   **Cooking time:** 25 minutes   **Portions: 3**

Ingredients:
- ½ tablespoon olive oil
- 2 tablespoons chopped onion
- 2 teaspoons of minced garlic
- ½ cup of carrots, peeled and chopped
- ½ cup of green cabbage, chopped
- 1/3 cup French beans, mashed

Directions:
- Heat the oil in a large heavy-bottomed frying pan over medium heat and fry the onion and garlic for about 4-5 minutes.
- Add the carrots, cabbage and beans and cook for about 4-5 minutes, stirring frequently.
- Stir in the broth and bring to the boil.
- Cook for about 4-5 minutes.

Ingredients:
- 3 cups of homemade vegetable stock
- ½ tablespoon fresh lemon juice
- 3 tablespoons of water
- 2 tablespoons arrowroot starch
- Sea salt and freshly ground black pepper, to taste

- Meanwhile, in a small bowl, dissolve the arrowroot starch in water.
- Slowly add the arrowroot starch mixture, stirring constantly.
- Cook for about 7-8 minutes, stirring occasionally.
- Add the lemon juice, salt and black pepper and remove from the heat.
- Serve hot.

190) Lentil and spinach soup

Preparation time: 15 minutes   **Cooking time:** 1¼ hours Total time: 1½ hoursPayments   **Portions: 6**

Ingredients:
- 2 tablespoons of olive oil
- 2 carrots, peeled and cut into pieces
- 2 stalks of celery, chopped
- 2 sweet onions, chopped
- 3 cloves of garlic, minced
- 1½ cups brown lentils, rinsed
- 2 cups of tomatoes, finely chopped
- ¼ teaspoon dried basil, crushed
- ¼ teaspoon dried oregano, crushed
- ¼ teaspoon dried thyme, crushed

Directions:
- In a large soup pot, heat the oil over medium heat and sauté the carrot, celery and onion for about 5 minutes.
- Add the garlic and fry for about 1 minute.
- Add the lentils and fry for about 3 minutes.
- Stir in the tomatoes, herbs, spices and stock and bring to the boil.

Ingredients:
- 1 teaspoon ground cumin
- ½ teaspoon ground coriander
- ½ teaspoon of paprika
- 6 cups of vegetable stock
- 3 cups fresh spinach, chopped
- Sea salt and freshly ground black pepper, to taste
- 2 tablespoons fresh lemon juice

- Reduce the heat to low and simmer, partially covered, for about 1 hour or until cooked to perfection.
- Add the spinach, salt and black pepper and cook for about 4 minutes.
- Add the lemon juice and remove from the heat.
- Serve hot.

191) Vegetarian stew

Preparation time: 20 minutes   **Cooking time:** 35 minutes   **Portions: 8**

Ingredients:
- 2 tablespoons of coconut oil
- 1 large sweet onion, chopped
- 1 medium parsnip, peeled and chopped
- 3 tablespoons of homemade tomato paste
- 2 large cloves of garlic, minced
- ½ teaspoon ground cinnamon
- ½ teaspoon ground ginger
- 1 teaspoon ground cumin
- ¼ teaspoon cayenne pepper

Directions:
- In a large soup pot, melt the coconut oil over medium-high heat and sauté the onion for about 5 minutes.
- Add the parsnips and fry for about 3 minutes.
- Stir in the tomato paste, garlic and spices and fry for about 2 minutes.

Ingredients:
- 2 medium-sized carrots, peeled and chopped
- 2 medium purple potatoes, peeled and cut into pieces
- 2 medium sweet potatoes, peeled and cut into pieces
- 4 cups of homemade vegetable stock
- 2 cups fresh cabbage, cut and chopped
- 2 tablespoons fresh lemon juice
- Sea salt and freshly ground black pepper, to taste

- Stir in the carrots, potatoes, sweet potatoes and stock and bring to the boil.
- Reduce the heat to medium-low and simmer covered for about 20 minutes.
- Add the cabbage, lemon juice, salt and black pepper and simmer for about 5 minutes.
- Serve hot.

SNACKs

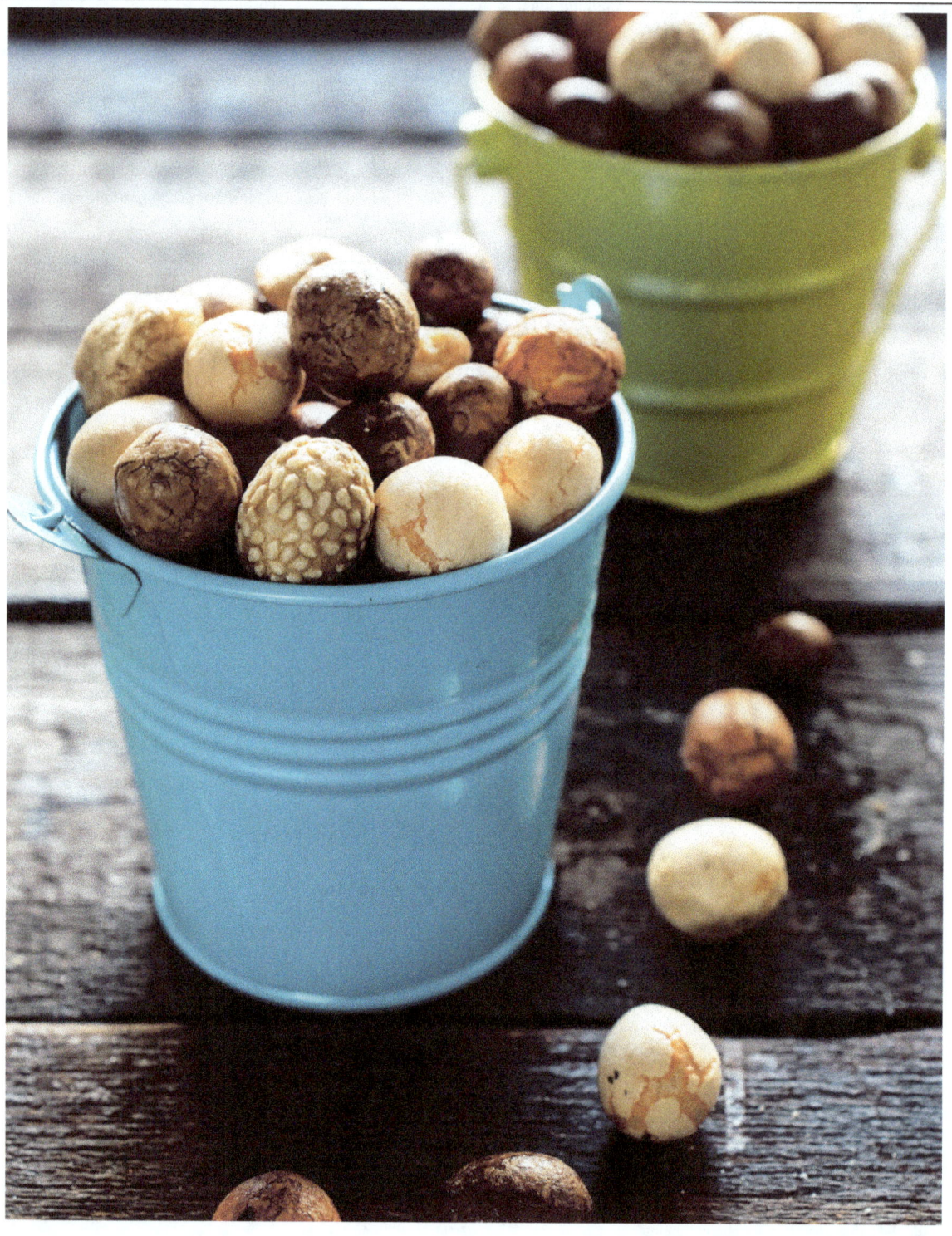

192) Alka-Goulash fast

Preparation time: **Cooking time:**   **Portions: 4**

Ingredients:
- 1 onion, finely chopped
- 1 clove of garlic, crushed
- 2 carrots, diced
- 3 courgettes, diced
- 2 tablespoons of olive oil
- 1 tablespoon paprika
- 1/4 teaspoon ground nutmeg

Ingredients:
- 1 tablespoon fresh parsley, chopped
- 1 tablespoon of tomato puree
- 2 cups tomatoes, peeled
- 2 cups of cooked, drained and rinsed red beans
- 1/2 cup of tomato juice
- Salt and black pepper to taste

Directions:
- Fry the onion, garlic, carrot and courgette in olive oil over a medium heat for 5 minutes, until softened.
- Add paprika, nutmeg, parsley and tomato puree.
- Add the tomatoes, red beans and tomato juice and mix.
- Simmer for 10 minutes until heated through.
- Serve immediately. Enjoy your meal!

193) Pea risotto

Preparation time: **Cooking time:**   **Portions: 4**

Ingredients:
- 1 vegetable stock cube
- 2 tablespoons of olive oil
- 1 onion, finely chopped
- 3 cloves of garlic, finely chopped
- 1 cup basmati rice

Ingredients:
- 1 cup frozen peas
- 1 cup of fresh spinach leaves
- 1 lemon, grated and squeezed
- Salt and black pepper to taste
- 3 cups of water

Directions:
- Crumble the vegetable stock cube into 3 cups of boiling water. Let it dissolve and then reduce the heat.
- Thaw the peas in hot water, drain them and set them aside for later.
- Season the onion with salt and black pepper to taste, and then fry in olive oil over medium heat for about 5 minutes, until softened.
- Add the garlic to the pan and fry it for a few minutes, taking care not to burn it.
- Add the rice to the pan and stir well. Pour in a little vegetable stock so that the rice is barely covered.
- Simmer over a medium heat, stirring constantly, for several minutes, until the liquid has been almost completely absorbed.
- Add the rest of the stock one ladle at a time, stirring constantly until each batch of stock has been absorbed.
- When each ladleful has been absorbed and the rice is fully cooked, add the defrosted peas, spinach leaves and lemon juice.
- Stir until the spinach leaves are wilted and serve hot.
- Have fun!

194) Satisfying lunch smoothie Alka

Preparation time: **Cooking time:**   **Portions: 1-2**

Ingredients:
- 1 large avocado
- 1.5 cup of coconut or almond milk
- 2 tablespoons of fresh coriander leaves
- 2 tablespoons of coconut oil

Ingredients:
- 1 lemon, squeezed
- 4 tablespoons of chia seeds
- Himalayan salt to taste

Directions:
- Simply blend all the ingredients except the seeds and oil.
- Stir well, add the chia seeds and enjoy with Himalayan salt.
- Have fun!

195) Alkaline pizza bread

Preparation time: **Cooking time:**   **Portions: 1**

Ingredients:
- Linseed, 100g
- Sunflower seeds, 200g
- Pepper, a pinch
- Dried tomatoes, 50g

Ingredients:
- Organic salt or sea salt, a pinch
- Extra virgin olive oil (cold pressed), 4 teaspoons
- Optional: Fresh wild garlic

Directions:
- Note: You need to soak the sunflower seeds for at least four hours.
- Blend the flax seeds in a blender until they are reduced to a powder.
- Once the sunflower seeds have lasted up to four hours, put them in a blender and blend them for a few seconds.
- Now add all the ingredients into a bowl.
- Using your hands, form a dough until it reaches the right consistency.
- The idea is to form a couple of pizza/bread crusts.
- Place them in a dehydrator or oven and dehydrate for up to twelve hours. Serve.

196) Alkaline-filled avocado

Preparation time: **Cooking time:**   **Portions:**

Ingredients:
- Oregano, 1 teaspoon
- Ripe avocado, 1
- Lime juice (fresh), 1 teaspoon
- Fresh basil, 1 teaspoon

Ingredients:
- Chopped onions, 1 teaspoon
- Tomato, ½
- Extra virgin olive oil (cold pressed), 4 teaspoons
- Pepper and sea salt

Directions:
- Cut the avocado into two equal halves and remove the seed.
- Use salt and pepper to season both halves.
- Mix the olive oil, chopped onion, lime juice and chopped tomato and put it in the holes of the avocado.
- Sprinkle with oregano and basil and serve.

197) Alkaline potato salad

Preparation time: **Cooking time:**   **Portions: 4**

Ingredients:
- Cauliflower, 1 cup
- Dill, 2 tablespoons
- Vegenaise, 1 teaspoon
- Red onion, 1
- Cucumber (small), 1
- Broccoli, 2 cups

Ingredients:
- Green/red pepper (small), 1
- Red potatoes, 600g
- Juice of 1 lemon
- Sea salt
- Olive oil (cold pressed), 3 tablespoons

Directions:
- Steam the cauliflower and broccoli for a few minutes and make sure they are crispy.
- Also, steam the potatoes until they are slightly soft and let them cool.
- Once they have cooled, slice the potatoes but do not remove the skin and throw them into a large bowl.
- Then, add the chopped cucumber, cauliflower, pepper, broccoli, dill, finely chopped onion and salt.
- Mix well and set aside.
- Take a small bowl and mix the veganaise, olive oil and lemon juice until smooth.
- Stir it into the potato salad and mix gently.
- It can be served immediately, but it is better to set it aside for a few hours (because it tastes better that way).
- You are free to add other seasonings according to your taste.

198) Almonds with sautéed vegetables

Preparation time: **Cooking time:** **Portions: 4**

Ingredients:
- Young beans, 150g
- Broccoli florets, 4
- Oregano and cumin, ½ teaspoon
- Lemon juice (fresh), 3 tablespoons
- Garlic clove (finely chopped), 1

Directions:
- Add the broccoli, beans and other vegetables to a large frying pan and fry until the beans and broccoli turn dark green.
- Make sure that the vegetables are also crispy.
- Now add the chopped garlic and onion, fry and stir for a few minutes.

Ingredients:
- Cauliflower, 1 cup
- Olive oil (cold pressed), 4 tablespoons
- Pepper and salt to taste
- Some soaked almonds (sliced), for garnish
- Yellow onion, 1
- Then, put the seasoning together.
- Take a small bowl, add the lemon juice, oregano, cumin and oil and mix well.
- Add some vegetables, stir slowly and taste for pepper and salt.
- Finally, use the sliced almonds as a garnish.
- Serve.

199) Alkaline sweet potato mash

Preparation time: **Cooking time:** **Portions: 3-4**

Ingredients:
- Sea salt, 1 tablespoon
- Curry powder, ½ table spoon
- Sweet potatoes (large), 6

Directions:
- First, take a large mixing bowl.
- Wash and cut the sweet potatoes and add them to the cooking pot and cook for about twenty minutes.

Ingredients:
- Coconut milk (fresh), 1 ½ - 2 cups
- Extra virgin olive oil (cold pressed), 1 tablespoon
- Pepper, 1 pinch
- Then, remove the sweet potatoes and mash them to the desired consistency.
- Finally, all you have to do is add the remaining ingredients and serve.

200) Mediterranean peppers

Preparation time: **Cooking time:** **Portions: 2**

Ingredients:
- Oregano, 1 teaspoon
- Garlic cloves (crushed), 2
- Fresh parsley (chopped), 2 tablespoons
- Vegetable bouillon (without yeast), 1 cup
- Provincial herbs, 1 teaspoon

Directions:
- Heat the olive oil in a frying pan over medium heat, add the pepper and onions and stir.
- Add the garlic and stir.

Ingredients:
- Red pepper (sliced) 2 + Yellow pepper (sliced) 2
- Red onions (thinly sliced), 2 medium-sized
- Extra virgin olive oil (cold pressed), 2 tablespoons
- Salt and pepper to taste
- Then, add the vegetable stock and season with parsley and herbs, as well as pepper and salt to taste.
- Cover the pan and leave to cook for fourteen to fifteen minutes.
- Serve.

201) Tomato and avocado sauce with potatoes

Preparation time: **Cooking time:** **Portions: 3**

Ingredients:
- Red onion 1
- 2 Tomatoes
- ½ - 1 lemon (squeezed)
- Chives (fresh and chopped), 1 teaspoon
- Parsley (fresh and chopped), 1 teaspoon

Directions:
- Take a pan and cook the potatoes in salted water, (cook the potatoes with the skin intact).
- Then, peel the avocado, throw it into a bowl and mash it with a fork.

Ingredients:
- Cayenne pepper, ½ teaspoon
- Avocado (ripe), 2
- Waxy potatoes (medium size), 6
- Saltwater
- Pepper and salt
- Now, dice the onion and tomatoes and add them to the bowl along with the parsley, chives and cayenne.
- Mix well and season with pepper, lemon juice and salt.
- Serve together with the potatoes.

202) Alkaline beans and coconut

Preparation time:
Cooking time:
Portions: 4

Ingredients:
- Ground cumin, ½ teaspoon
- Red chilli pepper (crushed), 1-2
- Coconut milk (fresh), 3 tablespoons
- Dry flaked coconut, 1 tablespoon
- Garlic (chopped), 2 cloves
- Cayenne pepper, 1 pinch

Ingredients:
- Sea salt, 1 pinch
- Extra virgin olive oil (cold pressed), 3 tablespoons
- Fresh herbs of your choice, 1 teaspoon
- One (1) pound of green beans, cut into 1-inch pieces
- Fresh ginger (chopped), ½ teaspoon

Directions:
- Heat the oil in a frying pan and add the beans, cumin, garlic, ginger and glaze and fry for about six minutes.
- Add the coconut flakes and oil and fry until the milk is fully cooked (this can take three or four minutes).
- Season with pepper, salt and herbs to taste. Serve.

203) Alkaline vegetable lasagne

Preparation time:
Cooking time:
Portions: 1

Ingredients:
- Parsley root, 1
- Leek (small), 1
- Radish (small), 1
- Corn salad, 1
- Tomatoes (large), 3
- Garlic, 1 clove

Ingredients:
- Avocado (soft), 2
- Lemon (squeezed), 1-2
- Rocket, 1
- Parsley (a few)
- Red pepper, 1

Directions:
- Take a blender and add the lemon juice, the garlic clove and the avocado.
- Cut the pepper into thin strips, cut the leek into thin rings and finely grate the parsley root and radish. When you have finished, mix everything with the avocado cream.
- We start with the first layer of the lasagne.
- Place the corn salad in a casserole dish, add the avocado spread well.
- For the second layer, add the sliced tomatoes.
- Finally, add the rocket and parsley for the final layer.
- Serve.

204) Aloo Gobi

Preparation time: **Cooking time:** **Servings: 1 bowl**

Ingredients:
- Cauliflower, 750g
- Fresh ginger, 20g
- Large onions, 2
- Mint, 1/3 cup
- Turmeric, 2 teaspoons
- Diced tomatoes, 400g
- Fresh garlic, 2 cloves
- Cayenne pepper, 2 teaspoons

Ingredients:
- Cilantro/coriander leaves, 1/3 cup
- Large potatoes, 4
- Garam masala, 2 teaspoons
- Green chilli, 4
- Water, 3 cups
- Extra virgin olive oil (cold pressed), 125 ml
- Salt to taste

Directions:
- Blend the chilli, garlic and ginger.
- Fry the oil in a wok for three minutes and add the onion until golden brown.
- Add the ground pasta and fry for a few seconds, then add; garam masala, chilli, turmeric, tomatoes and salt.
- Cook for about five minutes and add all the other ingredients.
- Stir for three minutes and add the water.
- Cook until the sauce is thick.
- Serve with Basmati rice or as a side dish.

DESSERTS

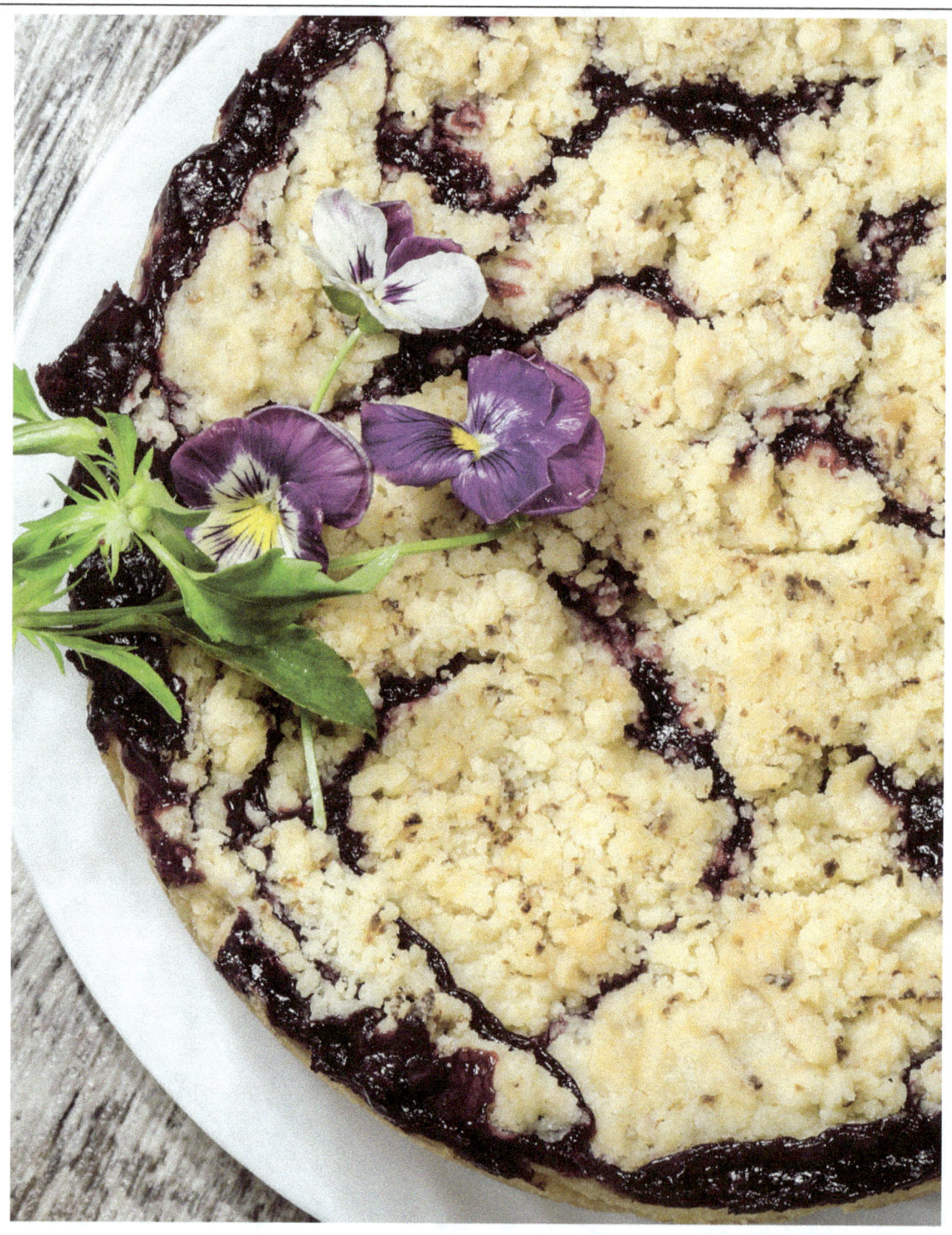

205) Pumpkin smoothie

Preparation time: 10 minutes   **Cooking time**:   **Portions**: 2

Ingredients:
- 1 cup of homemade pumpkin puree
- 1 medium banana, peeled and sliced
- 1 tablespoon maple syrup
- 1 teaspoon ground linseed

Directions:
- Place all ingredients in a high-speed blender and pulse until creamy.

Ingredients:
- ½ teaspoon ground cinnamon
- ¼ teaspoon ground ginger
- 1½ cups unsweetened almond milk
- ¼ cup ice cubes
- Pour the smoothie into two glasses and serve immediately.

206) Red fruit and vegetable smoothie

Preparation time: 10 minutes **Cooking time:** **Portions:** 2

Ingredients:
- ½ cup of fresh raspberries
- ½ cup of fresh strawberries
- ½ red pepper, seeded and chopped
- ½ cup red cabbage, chopped

Directions:
- Place all ingredients in a high-speed blender and pulse until creamy.

Ingredients:
- 1 small tomato
- 1 cup of water
- ½ cup of ice cubes

- Pour the smoothie into two glasses and serve immediately.

207) Kale smoothie

Preparation time: 10 minutes **Cooking time:** **Portions:** 2

Ingredients:
- 3 fresh cabbage stalks, cut and chopped
- 1-2 celery stalks, chopped
- ½ avocado, peeled, pitted and chopped

Directions:
- Place all ingredients in a high-speed blender and pulse until creamy.

Ingredients:
- ½ inch ginger root, chopped
- ½ inch turmeric root, chopped
- 2 cups of coconut milk

- Pour the smoothie into two glasses and serve immediately.

208) Green tofu smoothie

Preparation time: 10 minutes **Cooking time:** **Portions:** 2

Ingredients:
- 1½ cups cucumber, peeled and roughly chopped
- 3 cups of fresh spinach
- 2 cups of frozen broccoli
- ½ cup of tofu silken, drained and pressed

Directions:
- Place all ingredients in a high-speed blender and pulse until creamy.

Ingredients:
- 1 tablespoon fresh lime juice
- 4-5 drops of liquid stevia
- 1 cup unsweetened almond milk
- ½ cup ice, crushed

- Pour the smoothie into two glasses and serve immediately.

209) Grape and chard smoothie

Preparation time: 10 minutes **Cooking time:** **Portions:** 2

Ingredients:
- 2 cups of seedless green grapes
- 2 cups fresh beets, cut and chopped
- 2 tablespoons maple syrup

Directions:
- Place all ingredients in a high-speed blender and pulse until creamy.

Ingredients:
- 1 teaspoon fresh lemon juice
- 1½ cups of water
- 4 ice cubes

- Pour the smoothie into two glasses and serve immediately.

210) Matcha Smoothie

Preparation time: 10 minutes **Cooking time**: **Portions**: 2

Ingredients:
- 2 tablespoons of chia seeds
- 2 teaspoons matcha green tea powder
- ½ teaspoon fresh lemon juice
- ½ teaspoon xanthan gum

Directions:
- Place all ingredients in a high-speed blender and pulse until creamy.

Ingredients:
- 8-10 drops of liquid stevia
- 4 tablespoons of coconut cream
- 1½ cups unsweetened almond milk
- ¼ cup ice cubes
- Pour the smoothie into two glasses and serve immediately.

211) Banana smoothie

Preparation time: 10 minutes **Cooking time**: **Portions**: 2

Ingredients:
- 2 cups of cooled unsweetened almond milk
- 1 large frozen banana, peeled and sliced

Directions:
- Place all ingredients in a high-speed blender and pulse until creamy.

Ingredients:
- 1 tablespoon almonds, chopped
- 1 teaspoon organic vanilla extract
- Pour the smoothie into two glasses and serve immediately.

212) Strawberry smoothie

Preparation time: 10 minutes **Cooking time**: **Portions**: 2

Ingredients:
- 2 cups of cooled unsweetened almond milk
- 1½ cups of frozen strawberries

Directions:
- Add all ingredients to a high-speed blender and pulse until smooth.

Ingredients:
- 1 banana, peeled and sliced
- ¼ teaspoon organic vanilla extract
- Pour the smoothie into two glasses and serve immediately.

213) Raspberry and tofu smoothie

Preparation time: 15 minutes **Cooking time**: **Portions**: 2

Ingredients:
- 1½ cups of fresh raspberries
- 6 ounces of hard boiled tofu silken, drained
- 1/8 teaspoon of coconut extract

Directions:
- Add all ingredients to a high-speed blender and pulse until smooth.

Ingredients:
- 1 teaspoon stevia powder
- 1½ cups unsweetened almond milk
- ¼ cup ice cubes, crushed
- Pour the smoothie into two glasses and serve immediately.

214) Mango smoothie

Preparation time: 10 minutes   **Cooking time**:   **Portions: 2**

Ingredients:
- 2 cups frozen mango, peeled, stoned and chopped
- ¼ cup almond butter
- Pinch of ground turmeric

Ingredients:
- 2 tablespoons fresh lemon juice
- 1¼ cup unsweetened almond milk
- ¼ cup ice cubes

Directions:
- Add all ingredients to a high-speed blender and pulse until smooth.
- Pour the smoothie into two glasses and serve immediately.

215) Pineapple smoothie

Preparation time: 10 minutes   **Cooking time**:   **Portions: 2**

Ingredients:
- 2 cups pineapple, chopped
- ½ teaspoon fresh ginger, peeled and chopped
- ½ teaspoon ground turmeric
- 1 teaspoon of natural immune support supplement*.

Ingredients:
- 1 teaspoon chia seeds
- 1½ cups of cold green tea
- ½ cup ice, crushed

Directions:
- Add all ingredients to a high-speed blender and pulse until smooth.
- Pour the smoothie into two glasses and serve immediately.

216) Cabbage and pineapple smoothie

Preparation time: 15 minutes   **Cooking time**:   **Portions: 2**

Ingredients:
- 1½ cups fresh cabbage, chopped and shredded
- 1 frozen banana, peeled and chopped
- ½ cup of fresh pineapple chunks

Ingredients:
- 1 cup unsweetened coconut milk
- ½ cup of fresh orange juice
- ½ cup of ice

Directions:
- Add all ingredients to a high-speed blender and pulse until smooth.
- Pour the smoothie into two glasses and serve immediately.

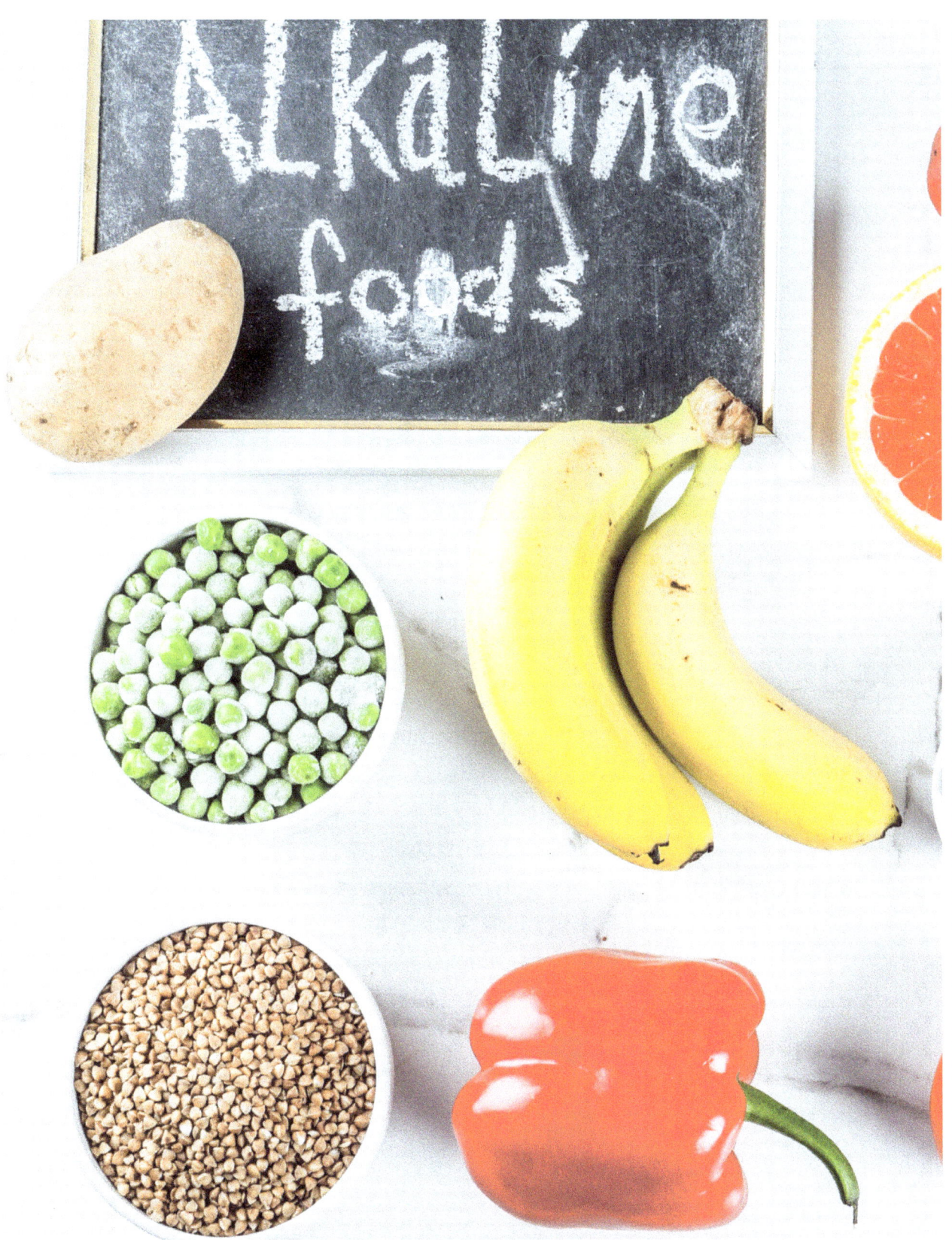

AUTHOR BIBLIOGRAPHY

THE ESSENCIAL ALKALINE DIET COOKBOOK FOR BEGINNERS

100+ Alkaline Recipes to Bring Your Body Back to Balance! Healthy Recipes to Enjoy Favorite Foods for Weight-Loss!

THE ALKAINE HEALTHY DIET FOR WOMEN

The Effective Way to Follow an Alkaline Diet comprising Plant-Based Diet Recipes: Natural Ways to Prevent Diabetes! 100+ Recipes Included!

THE ALKAINE HEALTHY DIET FOR MEN

100+ Recipes to Understand pH, Eat Well, and Reclaim Your Health! Plant-Based Recipes Are Included! Boost your Weight-Loss!

THE ALKAINE HEALTHY DIET FOR KIDS

100+ Recipes for Your Health, To Lose Weight Naturally and Bring Your Body Back to Balance

THE ALKALINE FIET COOKBOOK FOR ONE

100+ Recipes to Lose Weight and Get the Benefits of an Alkaline Diet - Alkaline Smoothies Included for Your Way to Vibrant Health - Massive Energy and Natural Weight Loss! Plant-Based Recipes Are Included!

THE ALKAINE DIET FOR WOMEN AFTER 50

2 Books in 1: The Complete Alkaline Diet Guidebook for Beginners: Understand pH, Eat Well with Easy Alkaline Diet Cookbook and more than 200+ Delicious Recipes (Lose weight, Beginners, Foods & Diet, Reset Cleanse)

THE SPECIAL ALKALINE DIET FOR TWO

2 Books in 1: Guidebook for Beginners: Understand pH, Eat Well with Easy Alkaline Diet Cookbook and more than 200 Delicious Recipes! Plant-Based Recipes Are Included!

THE ALKALINE DIET FOR DADDY AND SON

2 Books in 1: For Beginners: The Ultimate Guide of Alkaline Herbal Medicine for permanent weight loss, Understand pH with 200+ Anti Inflammatory Recipes Cookbook! Plant-Based Recipes Are Included!

THE ALKALINE DIET FAST & EASY

2 Books in 1: The Complete and Exhaustive Beginner's Guide to lose Weight, Fasting and Revitalize Your Body with Plant-Based Diet including 200+ Healthy and Tasty Recipes!

THE ALKALINE DIET FOR MUM AND KIDDOS

2 Books in 1: The Simplest Alkaline Diet Guide for Beginners + 200 Easy Recipes: How to Cure Your Body, Lose Weight and Regain Your Life with Easy Alkaline Diet Cookbook! Plant-Based Recipes Are Included!

THE ALKALINE DIET TO LOSE WEIGHT FAST

3 Books in 1: The Revolution of Eating Habits to stay Healthy and Find the Best Shape. A complete Program with 300+ Recipes to Regain a Healthy Balance of the Body with Alkaline Foods and lose Weight Quickly.

THE ALKALINE DIET FOR A HEALTHY FAMILY

3 Books in 1: A Complete Guide for Beginners to Clean and Treat Your Body, Eat Well with More Than 300+ Easy Alkaline Recipes for Weight Loss and Fight Chronic Disease!

THE ALKALINE DIET HIGH-PROTEIN FOR SPORT PLAYERS

3 Books in 1: Diet for Beginners: Top 300+ Alkaline Recipes for Weight Loss with Plant Based Diet And 21 Secrets To Reset And Understand pH Right Now!

THE ALKALINE DIET FOR ABSOLUTE BEGINNERS

3 Books in 1: This Cookbook Includes: Alkaline Diet for Beginners + Alkaline Diet Cookbook, The Best Guidebook to Understanding pH Secrets with More Than 300+ Recipes for Weight Loss and Anti-Inflammatory Action!

THE ALKALINE DIET COMPLETE EDITION FOR EVERYBODY

4 Books in 1: The complete guide to eat well and Lose Weight while understanding pH and prevent disease to boost your everyday energy! 400+ Recipes with Plant-Based Recipes Included!

CONCLUSIONS

Congratulations! You made it to the end!

Thank you for making it to the end of the Alkaline Diet; we hope it was informative and provided all you need to reach your goals, whatever they may be.

With the information you have, you can now start a successful alkaline diet. Your body works best when it's not acidic. The alkaline diet ensures that your body functions at its best. The great thing is that all the food you can eat is tasty. With the recipes in this book, you won't have to worry about making dinner. So don't wait any longer.

Start today, and you will see your body change for the better.

The purpose of this cookbook was to introduce readers to most of the insights regarding the alkaline diet in a comprehensive way. Therefore, the text of this book has been categorized into several sections, each of which discusses the basics, the details, what it has and what it doesn't, and recipes related to the alkaline diet. In addition, the recipe chapter is divided into subsections, ranging from breakfast to lunch, dinner, smoothies, snacks, and desserts. So take some time to travel the length of this book and experience the miraculous effects of an alkaline diet on your mind and health.

Laura Green

www.ingramcontent.com/pod-product-compliance
Lightning Source LLC
Chambersburg PA
CBHW081418080526
44589CB00016B/2583